The Alkaline Diet Plan Program:

The Best Selling Diet Book on How to Lose Weight with the Alkaline Water and Diet Plan with the Alkaline Diet Recipe Cookbook including Alkaline Diet Food and Juicing Recipes

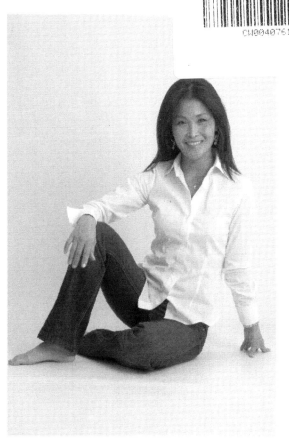

www.MyAlkalineDietPlan.com

By Dr. Connie Jeon

Doctor Physical Therapy
Masters Public Health, Nutrition
Baccalaureate Psychology
PMA Certified Pilates Instructor
Health-Fitness Specialist-ACSM
Certified Yoga Therapist
Macrobiotic Counselor
Registered Dietician

Table of Contents

Dedication

I dedicate this book to my wonderful husband and soul mate, Dr. Philip Jeon. Thank you for your support and faith in me.

Thank you to Jenny and Jay Cheung, my loving parents who's love has enabled me to newer heights.

I love you Brandon and Dylan, the greatest gifts from God.

My Journey

It took a long time for me to be clear about the content of my book. I had to take a long look at my life and the way events of my life shaped me before I can muster up the courage to share my knowledge and perspective with you. In the process I realized that while my education has served me well, it really restricted me and my creative thought process. It kept me from thinking on my own terms because I learned mostly theory and was trying to fit all my clinical and intuitive knowledge into the realm of my "learned knowledge" that the real extracted meaning the I myself have gathered were completely dismissed with the assumption that my views are well, just my views. What I found was that my views, direct experience, and perspective is what you would benefit from. My intention is not to throw another informational book to you, but provide you with the real life approach and the practical applications that you can really begin to use to recognize, remove, replenish, repeat, and restore your mind, body, and spirit. This I call the 5 R Matrix Implementation.

I've filtered through vast amount of research in various areas of medicine, nutrition, physical therapy, healing, eastern medicine, energy, and also the practical information that I gathered clinically, which allowed me to prove the benefits of my work through my patients. My back ground in the three aspects of discipline, psychology, nutrition, and physical therapy has really helped me to integrate and expand beyond the theory. I was able to thoroughly expand on the essence of mind, body, spirit connection and found that indeed there exists an amazing intercept of all three. Most importantly, that once cannot exist without the other.

It is important to recognize the three periods of our lives where we learn to create our values that will guide us the rest of our lives.

Imprint Period

The first period is the imprint period from birth to age 7. During the imprint period, we have very few filters, and whatever occurs gets imprinted very easily, at this phase, we are like a sponge taking in whatever information with virtually no filtering process.

Modeling Period

The second period is the modeling period, from age 7-14. During the modeling period, a child makes a choice about who to model. This is the period of hero-worship, where the kids idolize parents, movie stars, teachers, older siblings, etc. They begin to adopt values from their heroes.

Socialization Period

The third period is the socialization period from age 14-21. During this period the young adult begins to adopt social, sexual, and personal values and you start to make choices about what is important to you.

The reason why this concept is mentioned here is that in the process of my putting this information for you, I needed to understand myself and really define the "why" for me to be clear and effective.

My personal imprint period is very foggy, however, I can only assume that the little girl lives inside me who is very scared and afraid because of some traumatic events in the early part of my life. There are cultural influences that are so ingrained in me, such as dietary patterns, eastern old wives folk tales of various healing methods, Buddhist traditional practices that were exposed to me at a very young age. When I immigrated to the United States, my daily health practices of eating home cooked meals, and Buddhist rituals were done away and replaced with my frequent stops to McDonalds and going to church on Sundays.

My health consciousness began as a teenager, I was an avid workout junkie since I was 16 years old, mainly to look good. I had much the same body image issues as any teenager and strived to be fit and thin.

Then during my college years I was trying to exercise and eat the right foods, I remember carrying around carrot sticks to and from classes and refrained from high fat foods. I enjoyed a real challenge when it came to exercise, it was a habit that I forced myself to form more for self control. I used to be up at the crack of dawn and running laps at the college campus every morning. I recall the fatigue that used to set on me after bouts of exercise, I just dismissed as something positive "no pain, no gain".

Then, I remember this one spring day, March' 1999, I was studying with my classmates out on the lawn of our campus, I was really itchy all over my body and as I scratched, I broke out into hives. My stress level was at its all time high, my nature is very high strung and type "A". I came home to my loft and my roommate, who was a nurse, took a look and said I needed intervention as I was having a reaction to something. I thought nothing of it and took some Benadryl and it went away.

The following weekend, I went snowboarding and as it was my first time, I fell a lot as I was learning to maneuver the snow board. Two days after this, I remember severe fatigue and I started to have rashes around my joints, elbow, fingers, hips, knees..., then my face. I went to dermatologist, infectious disease doctors, internal medicine specialist, etc. and they could not figure it out, they said it was likely a reaction to something, this something being anything in the environment. This was not a satisfying answer as I was desperate to look and feel like myself again.

I was quite alarmed when I noticed that I was losing extreme amount of hair, it got to a point where I was noticing patches of baldness. I remember praying...."please God, you can take away everything, just leave my hair alone". I smile at the extent of my vanity now but at the time, it was far from being funny. My brother, who is a chiropractor, suspected that it was Lupus and wanted to run some tests, and confirmed that all lab profile matched with systemic Lupus. I then took the lab results to the rheumatologist and was officially diagnosed. Little did I know that I should've secured a healthcare plan prior to this diagnosis as my rheumatologist informed me that it'll be a challenge to get health coverage. Although I was in a doctoral program in Physical Therapy, I despondently believed that I was not going to be able to perform at my job. I was slowing dying at this time, giving up on all my hopes and ambitions I had in becoming a physical therapist, and setting up my successful practice that would grow into an empire.

I became very frail, I was losing weight drastically and felt extremely tired. I did not want anybody to know about my condition and I tried to cover all signs and symptoms of my condition, especially the malar rash on my face as well as the rashes on my hands that made me feel like I was infected with leprosy. I remember reading the story of Job in the Bible and wondering what God's purpose for me was. I managed to get through the last year of my doctoral studies, and during this time met my husband. I was going in and out of the hospital for mysterious fevers, projectile vomiting, tremors, pain, and severe headaches and the doctors diagnosed me with UTI (urinary tract infection), meningitis, and just shrugged their shoulders and assumed that it was all due to my Lupus and dismissed me with various medications, including antibiotics, prednisone, and narcotics.

This was the time when I wanted more answers. Although I was studying western medical philosophy, I became very curious about eastern medicine when my father advised that I see the oriental medicine doctor in Los Angeles who was on the Korean radio talking about Lupus. He claimed that he can cure Lupus. I went to see him and he regarded me, felt my pulse, had me lying down and palpated my organs. He told me the years of me being a vegetarian did not serve me, that I was extremely hypertensive with diminishing energy flow. He recommended that I meditate daily with breathing and take the herbal tea that he would prescribe for six months minimum three times a day. He also advised that I eat meat, that my body type would benefit from the proteins in the meat. Having studied nutrition at a Seventh Day Adventist Institution, I was a strict vegan for 5 years. I was skeptical because I believed that being a vegan was the only way to longevity and health.

I reluctantly agreed as I knew that no one would or can help me. I felt this would be my last opportunity. I kept this a secret from my rheumatologist, who said that Lupus is like a fire inside of me, once it starts to burn and destroy, it's difficult to contain, that his goal was to "contain" the fire and keep it simmering with corticosteroids.

Knowing what I know about the harm of corticosteroids, (mostly the vain effects of moon face, thinning of hair, and weight gain), I fought him to be at the lowest possible dose. Besides, keeping my disease "simmering" did not make sense, I wanted to get rid of the disease all together.

After 6 months of herbal tea, eating meat, and breathing, my antibody profile was at its best, the markers were substantially lower and my doctor was quizzically happy about it. I never did tell him what I was doing outside his intervention. My health was slowly being restored, I had fatigue at times but I never attributed it to Lupus and fought to keep my disease under control.

I had two healthy boys since then and had two severe kidney inflammation that almost took my life, however, with continued faith, practice in yoga/Pilates/qi gong, proper nutrition, stress control, and meditation, I am proud to say that today, my health is maintained with just vitamins, supplements, energetic healing methods, and meditation.

My vision is to help as many people as possible, giving them hope and courage to take control of their health and life, especially the ones that are suffering. I've committed to continued education in acupuncture, Qi Gong, Eastern Medicine, Visceral Mobilization, Manual Therapy, Functional Medicine/Nutrition, Yoga, Healing, Energy Medicine, Women's Health, and Pilates.

I've since founded and operated Novo Total Wellness from 2006-2011. I've given this business my heart and soul and found that my health deteriorated from the added stress. In my efforts to better manage my life, health, family, career balance, I've been on a sabbatical for the past year creating programs, writing, publishing, blogging, researching, and most importantly, being a mom and a wife to my adorable boys and my dear husband.

My goal is to help as many individuals by bringing them back to the basics and guiding them back to themselves. More people are suffering from mysterious ailments that are threatening the quality of their lives. This means that their health is below the threshold of "Dis-ease", as I once was. Imbalances in our internal and external "systems" breeds "Dis-ease", we must learn how to optimally keep our bodies at "ease" to live a life of abundance. I thank you for allowing me to share my knowledge and assist in your health.

Connie Jeon

The Transformation

I grew up in South Korea from birth to 10 years of age. The culture in Korea is fundamentally more spiritual. I remember Jesa, a ritual or a memorial to the deceased elders in the family, mainly ancestors of typically two generations. To perform ancestor rituals, the family at the eldest son's house prepare many kinds of food such as wine, taro soup, beef, fish, three different colored vegetables, many kinds of fruits, and rice cake or song pyon, particularly those that were favored by the deceased. The shinwi (신위, 神位) or memorial tablet, which symbolizes the spiritual presence of the ancestor, is placed at the center of the table. In modern days, the daughter or younger son of the family may perform these rites.

After midnight or in the evening before an ancestor's death anniversary, the descendants set the shrine, with a paper screen facing north and food laid out on a lacquer table as follows: rice, meat, and white fruits on the west, soup, fish, and red fruits on the east, with fruits on the first row, meat and fish on the second, vegetables on the third, and cooked rice and soup on the last. The rice bowls and individual offerings to the male ancestors are placed to the west, and those of females to the east (고서비동, 考西妣東). Two candles are also laid on both ends of the table, and an incense holder is placed in the middle. Every year, I would observe my family performing this memorial.

Since my family were Buddhists, I remember also going to the temple every so often and observe my parents and grandparents performing rituals, praying, bowing, and meditating.

One other practice that the elders in my family is relying on fortune telling. Fortune telling is very common in Korea, some fortune tellers utilize the facial features of an individual, birth time and date, their Korean name. My mom used to tell me that she's planned her c-section to have each and every one of us at a certain time and date and tried to give me this input when I was giving birth to my boys. My mother in law also sought a fortune teller to see if the marriage between my husband and me was suitable. This used to be so farfetched but as I learn more about the eastern medicine history, it fascinates me.

When I got sick with Lupus, the only thing that I can think about is what went wrong. I was obviously a health nut, exercising daily and eating a diet full of vegetables and fruits. Even as a scholar, the field of nutrition is very confusing. It's the once topic that everyone can relate to as we all have to eat. Many diet theories try to vary the food compositions between carbohydrates, fats, to protein. For example, the Atkins diet was all about the protein rich food, Jenny Craig is all about counting the carbs in meals, and the South beach diet is somewhere in the middle.

It was a slap in the face when of all the people with bad dietary practices around me, I was the one with diagnosed with Lupus. It upset and embarrassed me. When I first went to see Dr. Kim in Los Angeles, he assessed me and let me know that my body type based on the organs, facial structure, and temperament, needs protein source from red meat. This really took a while for me to digest because I was taught that vegetarian diet was be all and end all to health and wellness.

He said not everyone is the same constitution, that I needed to supply my body rich protein specifically from lean red meats. This was because my energetic level due to the dominant organ, specifically the liver that I would thrive on a high protein diet. This is when I learned that biochemical individuality need to be respected. I studied and followed Dr. Kim's guidance, however, I lost touch with him because I relocated to Georgia, which was 10 years ago.

I recently became very interested in the eastern medicine philosophy because I met a doctor, Dr. Chung, who contacted me and asked if he can treat and cure me of my condition (systemic Lupus) here in Georgia. It was when I was on a sabbatical and he was taking over the clinic that I was occupying. He wanted to contribute to my work as well as treat me in the hopes of working with me.

Despite my reluctance, he kept keeping in touch with me and asked me to come and experience his techniques, that he would treat me for free for as long as he can cure me. After feeling rather depleted due to my abdominal hernia repair in Oct 2011and suffering from a bout of IBS (irritable bowel syndrome) for the past year due to the stress from the business, I agreed. At this time, I also had severe melasma around the face, which was a pressing issue, I tried facials for 8 months with very little improvement. The first thing he did was examined my pulse and looked at my eyes and he told me the following:

1. I am very intelligent and very impatient.

2. I have very little vital energy left in me, that my gut was in terrible disharmony from all the stress and mechanical disruption from the surgery.

3. My body type is So Yang and that explains the temperament and my body shape.

4. I have very weak kidney energy and need to enhance the energetic forces.

5. As for my Lupus, that in western medicine, it's very difficult, that they can only chase the symptoms but in eastern medicine, it's very easy.

I was intrigued but it takes a lot for me to trust anyone, so I decided that I would try this out, after all, it was free. The first session, he said that he needed to treat the gut, which is the most important, (I agreed with this as in Functional Medicine, we learned that this was the first place to start with any patients.) He carefully inserted the needles in various places in my abdomen and attached wires that would transmit electrical impulses to get my energy to flow through the meridian channels that connect to my internal organs and when he turned on the machine, I can feel my gut moving with the rhythm, felt like peristalsis, which is the muscular contractions of the gut that allow food to pass and enables you to void the excess. It felt strange but good at the same time because I have not felt the movement in so long. I had a soft lump the size of a golf ball in my abdomen from the lack of energy flow as he described, I knew this was true because I've been terribly constipated since the surgery. After 10 months of acupuncture treatment, I can honestly say that my IBS is no longer a problem, I have no constipation, and I feel so much better.

I was both intrigued and curious, and I began to ask him questions every time I was there. He explained the five elements.

The Elements

There are five categories of elements in the natural universe. They are; wood, fire, earth, metal, and water. The traditional Chinese Medicine holds that all natural phenomena in the universe correspond in nature either to wood, fire, earth, metal, or water, and these elements are in constant motion and change. The theory of the five elements was first introduced in China at the time of the Yin and Zhou dynasties 16th century-221 B.C.). This is historically derived from observations that wood, fire, earth, metal, and water were considered to be five indispensable materials for the maintenance of life and production. Water and fire is essential for food and metal and wood are essential for production of goods, and earth gives life to everything.

What I found interesting was how it links the universal energy that exist in earth correspond in the same way in our bodies.

The elements correspond to different internal organs and the five elements are associated with the four seasons and the five tastes.

The five elements complement each other and react to each other. It is more accurate to understand the Five Elements theory as the Five Transformations or Five Phases.

The Five Elements theory views the Universe and its function as being cyclical and interactive. Accordingly, all of the things that exist in the universe are interdependent.

Chinese physicians and sages determined that each element had special relations with particular organs in the human body as well as to other characteristics such as colors, flavors, the time of day, the season of the year, and the way we respond physically and emotionally to external influences and the forces of nature.

The Five Elements theory identifies the five different modes (elements) in which qi energy manifest itself. The five elements (Wood, Fire, Earth, Metal and Water) are arranged into a cyclical sequence that represents the flow of energy between these elements as 'phases' in this specific sequence.

Each phase of an element characterizes a stage in a cyclical process.

The five elements theory is simply an observation on natural changes; everything can be in constant and harmonious transition from one phase to another - just as one season 'becomes' the next.

WOOD

Wood is considered the most human of all the elements. It is the element of spring, which is associated with the capacity to look forward, plan and make decisions. Wood energy is rising, expanding, and is the force of growth and flexibility.

This element represents all the activities of the body that are self regulating and/or function without conscious thought; i.e. digestion, respiration, heart beat and basic metabolism.

The liver (which converts food into fuel which is then supplied to the muscles, tendons and ligaments) is associated to the Wood element.

FIRE

Fire is the element of heat, summer, and enthusiasm; nature at its peak of growth, and warmth in human relationships. Its primary motion is upward. Fire is considered the symbolic of combustion which represents the functions of the body that have reached that threshold of maximum activity; indicating that decline is inevitable. The element is associated with the heart and related to the tongue.

EARTH

Earth is the element of harvest time, abundance, nourishment, fertility, and is likened to mother and child relationship. This element is also regarded as the center point of balance and the place where energy becomes downward in movement. It is the symbol of stability and being properly anchored.

Earth element is associated to the spleen and related to the sense of taste.

METAL

The metal element has the force of gravity, the minerals within the earth, and the powers of electrical conductivity and its magnetic nature. Metal has structure, but it can also accept a new form when molten with heat. Metal energy is consolidating and the movement tends to be inward, like a flower closing its petals. The characteristic of the metal element is one of a cutting and reforming action, but it also has the tendency to solidify. This element is associated with the lungs and associated to the nose.

WATER

Water is the source of life on this planet. Likewise it is the fluids (the main component of the body), which nourish and maintain the health of every cell. Water is vital to the body, forming vital fluids, i.e. blood, lymph, mucus, semen and fat. The kidney is especially linked to this element and its motion tend to be downward. Water has the capacity to flow, infinitely yielding and infinitely powerful, ever changing and has the capacity to nourish and cleanse.

Water is the ultimate yin; quiet and cold; representing the hibernation of winter. It has a patient, silent; still quality that considered as the "stored potential". It has flexibility (think of water filling up any shape of vessel), yet it has great power (think of the devastation caused by floods). In human psychology, the water element governs the balance between fear and the desire to dominate.

	Wood	**Fire**	**Earth**	**Metal**	**Water**
Organs	Liver/Gallbladder	Heart/Small Intestine	Stomach/Spleen	Lung/Large Intestine	Kidney/Bladder
Tastes	Sharp	Sweet	Sour	Bitter	Salty
Season	Spring	Summer		Sprint	Winter

Characteristics

According to the 5 Elements theory your internal organs, tissues, other parts of the body and their associated activities, all correspond to one or another as the Five Elements (phases). In healthy people, the elements are said to be balanced and in sick people they are said to be unbalanced. Indications of an imbalance may appear as various symptoms such as rash, pain, fever, mood swings, fatigue, etc.

The characteristic of each phase (yang to yin) is determined by the smooth phases of the seasons, the transition from one season to the next and how smoothly this occurs.

It is essential to eat a balanced diet which corresponds to the seasons, exercise moderately, and learn to manage and balance stress according to this theory. It is when we do not honor the natural changes of nature that our bodies become imbalanced and results in Disease.

The Alkaline Program
Introduction

There are so much information on diets, from Paleo Diet, Macrobiotic Diet, Atkins Diet, Jenny Craig, Westin A Price, South Beach Diet, Alkaline Diet, Raw Diet........Yikes, as a learned professional in the field of nutrition, it is confusing even for me! With so much information pouring in from everywhere and its availability with a click of a button you really need to be an informed consumer and learner. I've researched the diets and their principles, studied the foundations of nutrition and know that you don't need another "DIET". Simply because Diets don't work.

The sacred act of eating has become an act of obsession, compulsion, and deprivation. Let's remember, foods nourish and supply us with the essential building blocks to live and flourish. The problem is not the food, but our mental "relationship" and the "internal perception" of food. The Alkaline program incorporates the whole mind, body, and spirit to redefine our relationship to ourselves by altering our "internal map" of reality. It is proven that the mind is the ultimate control center for our behavior and desires. The answer lies in this very fact, if we can control our "control center" by reprogramming our internal map from disharmony with the universe to harmony with the universe, I am confident that you will never have to diet again.

Once the "control center" is reprogrammed, then we'll talk about altering behaviors such as eating, exercise/movement, and our internal thoughts to work with our goals rather than work against it. You see, if our mind does not perceive the benefits or the possibilities of what you are trying to accomplish, no matter how hard you try, by way of will power, you won't succeed. This is the very reason that diets do not work.

The goal of the Alkaline Program is to provide you with a comprehensive yet simplified approach to foster optimal health and wellness. I felt the need for a program that encompass the whole body, mind and spirit to really make the permanent changes necessary to stay on target of life of abundance, health, and happiness.

Our body is nothing short of a miraculous. It consists of the core energetic life force (QI) that sets the motion for its ability to heal, maintain homeostasis, evolve, and change. It is important to understand that its natural state is to be at its optimal health. The Modern American Lifestyle (MAL) is not conducive to maintaining the proper physiological, psychological, and spiritual balance to keep the body at a state of harmony both internally and externally. We are created to be one with the universe, however, the current conditions are altered so much from its natural state that our bodies are ever so challenged to keep its internal balance.

The Modern American Lifestyle consists of poor diet, increased stress, lack of movement, and lack of consciousness, which ultimately results in disharmony. The Modern American Diet (MAD) is full of refined foods, additives, GMO (genetically modified), hormones/antibiotics (live stocks), toxins, lack of vegetables and fruits, and it's getting worse. The stress is at its peak with information overload, increased demands at work, lack of time, poor economic conditions, with no signs of improvement in the near future makes the stress levels at its peak and beyond. To add to this, we are fasting from exercise or movement due to the increased weight, lack of motivation, fatigue, and various joint or muscle pains. The Alkaline Program has a complete solution for you to transform your health, lose weight, find happiness, harmony, balance, improve energy, memory, and be pain free.

The Alkaline program has three parts; The Alkaline Mind, Alkaline Abs (Physiology), and the Alkaline Dieting. These three parts make up the whole body system that will allow you to really address the foundation of your health and tackle all components so that the transformation is permanent. Each part consist of the 5R matrix implementation system that will guide your process;

RECOGNIZE - Awareness, Identify the core of the problem, learn to recognize and notice it.

REMOVE - Detox old habits, MAD diet, negative thoughts, bad posture, dysfunctional movement patterns, negative thinking patterns, and physical imbalances

REPLENISH/REPROGRAM - Replenish with the right probiotics, foods, learn proper posture, learn new behaviors and instill positive thoughts that will guarantee results.

REPEAT/RECONNECT - Affirmations, meditations, guided imagery, reinforcement - FORMING NEW HABITS that are permanent. Don't let setbacks discourage you, keep looking forward.

RESTORE/RESTART-- restore the desired behaviors and if you get off track, then restart the 5 R matrix system.

Part I:
The Alkaline Mind

Romans 12:2 ESV

Do not be conformed to this world, but be transformed by the renewal of your mind, that by testing you may discern what is the will of God, what is good and acceptable and perfect.

The Alkaline program is effective because it addresses the mind, body, spirit. We know that will power to change the way we eat is not effective, we snap back to our old habits just as the rubber band snaps back to its original form when stretched. This is because our internal programming from birth is ingrained mostly in the subconscious mind. No matter how hard we consciously "try" to change our habits, we are at a tremendous disadvantage if we do not make a change at the subconscious level.

The computer between our two ears has tremendous potential but we need to learn to tap into the subconscious. The healing power reside in the mind. So how can we use this knowledge to change the pH of our physiology?

As I mentioned in the prior articles, the Modern American Lifestyle is one that promotes stress, sleep deprivation, sedentary life, negative thoughts, and poor diet. We know that despite the current perceptual conditions around you, your thoughts dictate your reality. It is important to note that your thoughts are energy and can influence your hormone secretion, biochemical enzymes, neurotransmitters, metabolic system, musculoskeletal system, and the immune system.

The stress response can trigger a immune response and create symptoms due to the above affects such as rash, indigestion, fatigue, pain, etc. In order for us to have abundance, health, and happiness, we need to think differently, especially if you don't have the aforementioned. Our program teaches you step by step how to make permanent changes that are so powerful that it'll positively influence your whole life, not just the "diet". Our body is whole being, not the sum of its parts, we need to address the whole being, not in parts.

The Alkaline Mind program will cover the basics of the brain and its parts. You will understand the workings of the brain and how it affects our physiology and behavioral patterns. You will also understand how your thoughts can dictate the quality of your life, how stressors alter the whole body systems that can cause disease states. You will learn to appreciate this amazing organ and more importantly, learn to utilize it to your benefit. You will also realize that you have no limits, only the ones you set for yourself. I welcome you into taking a deeper look at what you are capable of.

Section 1:
Brain Basics

Your brain is the master of your soul, it dictates the essence of your being and therefore define who you really are. Your brain can affect the way you feel, how you interact with others, and it can affect your behavior. The physiology of your brain can cause anxiety, depression, obsessive-compulsive disorders, ADHD (attention deficit disorder), autism, anger, etc. The brain can also make you more prone to diseases by way of neurotransmitters that can impact your immune system and cause a cascade of hormonal disorders that can lead to many different symptoms that can be devastating.

We've come a long way into really understanding how our brains function. Your brain contains 100 billion nerve cells that constantly form trillion to quadrillion connections called synapses. These connections allow you to be dynamic by remodeling and adapting to the world around you. It is no wonder that we stand in reverence and in awe of the brain because not only is it capable of interpretation of the world around you, but it is capable of creating the world for you. It can interpret so much information at once, including what you hear, see, feel, touch, taste, and smell.

Until recently, researchers can only speculate the brain's role in personality traits, however, currently have advanced tools to prove that the brain can affect behaviors, from relationships, career, and ultimately the essence of an individual.

What we do know about the brain is that the physiology of the brain can also be altered that can have a better outcome both in behavior and attitude. This is great news for many of us who are suffering from various forms of disorders including Alzheimer's, ADHD, Autism, OCD, anxiety, and depression. In fact, what I am about to share with you in the Alkaline Mind will allow you to tap into the infinite possibilities of your brain, that you already possess. It's been said that the majority of the people only utilize up to 10 % of our full brain potential. We tend to succumb to the status quo, and tend to become set in our habits and behaviors. For example, we tend to perform the same tasks, eat the same foods, and enjoy the same activities day in and day out. It's very disturbing when we try to change our routines (for most of us) because our neural programming is set and it is difficult to adapt to the new behaviors and habits unless we are determined to change. A great example is the efforts that most of us put forth into losing weight. This takes tremendous effort and as a rubber band when stretched out to its max and let go, it snaps back into its original form and shape. However, there is a better way to adapt new behaviors such as exercise and healthy eating habits by reprogramming your brain, which I will be sharing with you.

Let's review how the brain activity is measured and how it can be used to understand the brain activity.

Brain waves are generated by the individual cells called neurons. Neurons communicate with each other by electrical changes. We can actually see these electrical changes in the form of brain waves as shown in an EEG (electroencephalogram). Brain waves are measured in cycles per second (Hertz; Hz is the short form). We also talk about the "frequency" of brain wave activity. The lower the frequency as measured in Hz, the slower the brain activity and conversely, the higher the frequency, the higher brain activity.

Researchers in the 1930's and 40's identified several different types of brain waves. Traditionally, these fall into 4 types:

- Delta waves (below 4 Hz) typically occur during sleep

- Theta waves (4-7 Hz) are associated with sleep, deep relaxation, and visualization

- Alpha waves (8-13 Hz) typically when we are relaxed and calm

- Beta waves (13-38 Hz) typically when we are actively thinking, problem-solving, etc.

- The Sensory motor rhythm (or SMR; around 14 Hz) was originally discovered to prevent seizure activity in cats. SMR activity seems to link brain and body functions.

- Gamma brain waves (39-100 Hz) are involved in higher mental activity and consolidation of information. This brain wave is most common with Tibetan monks who's been practicing meditation for years.

It is important to note that we don't ever produce only "one" brain wave type. Our overall brain activity is a mix of all the frequencies concurrently, some dominating in quantity and strength than others.

What does this mean for you? That it is important to produce dynamic balance of this brain wave patterns. How do we do this? I will go over the brain and its functions section by section and will give you an implementation guide organized in the 5 R Matrix system.

It is important to remain flexible, which generally means being able to shift ideas or actions to get optimal results.

We need to be able to shift our brain activity to match what we are doing. At work, we need to stay focused and attentive and those beta waves are a Good Thing. But when we get home and want to relax, we want to be able to produce less beta and more alpha activity. To get to sleep, we want to be able to decrease the brain wave pattern even more.

We also have difficulty when we get stuck in a certain pattern. One is more susceptible after injury of some kind to the brain (which can be physical or emotional), the brain tries to heal itself and it slows down. however, if the brain stays that slow, if it gets "stuck" in the slower frequencies, you will have difficulty concentrating and focusing, thinking clearly, etc. For example, when you are driving, you need to be able to speed up to the limit on the highway and slow down when driving behind the school bus. If you drive slowly at the highways and fast at the stop light, it can be devastating.

So flexibility is a key goal for efficient brain functioning.

Resilience means stability - being able to bounce back from stressors or negative events and to "bend with the wind, not break". Studies show that people who are resilient are healthier and happier than those who are not.

Same thing in the brain. The brain needs to be able to "bounce back" from all the stressors that we impose on to it (drinking, smoking, falling, accidents, etc.) The resilience we need to stay healthy and happy resides in the brain.

What are the insults that cause our brains to be dysfunctional? Head injury, medications, alcohol, drugs, fatigue, emotional stress, and general stress.

In the following sections we will go over each system of our brain and understand the functions of each system. Then at the end of each section I've provided the 5 R Matrix implementation system that is easy to follow so that you can begin to use and make changes immediately. Remember, our brain and our mind is the ultimate control center for all else. If we can master our mind and brain, we can achieve anything.

Section 2:
The Limbic System

The limbic system lies near the center of the brain. It's about the size of a walnut and it is power packed with functions that are essential for human behavior and survival. The limbic system is considered the older part of the mammalian brain that allowed animals to express their emotions.

The limbic system is responsible for setting the emotional tone for the day. If you are sad, it means you have an overactive limbic system and the events through the day will likely seem negative to you. However, when the limbic system is working properly, the events during the day may seem more neutral or positive. This is important for behavior because negative interpretation will cause us to avoid the situation and the positive interpretation will drive us to action.

The limbic system tend to store highly charged emotional events in life, both positive and negative. The cumulative experiences of our life is partly responsible for the emotional tendencies of our mind. More traumatic events we have, will cause us to be more withdrawn full of fear and the more positive experiences that we have, the more proactive our tendencies.

The Limbic system is also responsible for sleep, appetite, and the social adaptability. It is also intimately connected to our sense of smell. It is no wonder that the smell can influence the emotional state of a person, including the sexual desires.

It is also important to note that the women tend to have larger limbic system than men, this explains why women tend to be more emotionally charged than men. Women are more expressive and are more in touch with their feelings than their counterparts. This leaves women more susceptible to depression, especially during times of hormonal fluctuations such as puberty, pre-menstrual, post partum, and menopause. The statistics are that the women are more suicidal by at least three times more than men.

Do you suspect that you or anyone you know have Limbic System disorder?

• Do you feel sad?

• Have low energy?

- Have mood swings?

- Feel hopeless?

- Suicidal thoughts?

- Cry for no reason?

- Low self esteem?

- Decreased Libido?

- Difficulty concentrating?

- Poor Memory?

Healing the Limbic System:

Due to the fact that the negative thoughts may be dominating your life, we need to alter the thought patterns from negative to positive. Did you know that your thoughts have a physiological impact in your body? They influence the cells by sending electrical impulses and carry energy. Learning how to observe your patterns and altering them to the positive thought pattern will allow you to feel better and heal the disorder of the limbic system. Yes, it's that easy.

I recommend a five R Matrix from the Alkaline Program: Follow the five R Matrix and you'll be on your way to healing your limbic system.

Recognize:

Take an assessment of your mind day in and day out. What self defeating thoughts run throughout the day? I'm not good enough, I'm just this way, I'm fat by nature, my life is horrible, I'm not good at _____ I'm not going to make it, it's too hard.

Do you tend to

- expect the worst in any situation?

- believe that other people are thinking negative thoughts about you when you don't know for sure?

- do you constantly think about what you should, ought, or have to do?

- do you take everything personally?

- blame and resent others for the negative events in your life?

count them and take note

Remove:

Any time you find yourself thinking negative thoughts or feelings, immediately flick the switch to the positive thought and feelings. Think the opposite of what you are thinking, and detach from whatever is happening. See if you can observe as a third person and advise yourself to remove those toxic thoughts and replace with positive ones.

It's also important to avoid those individuals that tend to be negative and not supportive for your efforts. We all have them in our lives, they may be your friends, co-workers, family, spouse, children. It's hard to remove those that are close to you, like your family, however, you can try to keep distance until you are reprogrammed and rewired to handle their negativity. Attitudes of others are contagious, so be selective in who you surround yourself with.

Remember that the sense of smell is directly related to the limbic system. Remove all odors that may be tampering with your moods, especially around the places that you spend most of your time, your bedroom, home, car, office, etc.

Remove all refined foods, additives, soda, juice, and sugar. Limit the intake of caffeinated drinks such as coffee and soda and alcoholic beverages.

Replenish/Reprogram

Immediately reprogram your mind to bypass the "automatic" thoughts or the programmed thoughts and flip switch the thought to the positive alternative and associate good "feelings" because emotions are what is key to the success of this.

You need to do this on a regular basis to be successful, where the mind goes, energy goes......use imagery of positive thoughts, goals, and beliefs.

Surround yourself with the people that support your efforts and those that make you feel good. There are people that are just pleasant to be around because they are always so happy and positive, make new friends and enjoy the new relationships.

Add some great scents that you like to the places that you spend ample amount of your time in. You'll see that this will greatly affect your limbic system and help it to heal faster.

Add physical movement daily. Regular movement releases endorphins that induce a sense of well being. Since the limbic system has ample amount of endorphin receptors, it can directly impact its healing. Regular physical movement will do wonders for clarity in thinking with increased blood circulation to the brain and the rest of the body, increased metabolic rate for weight loss and control, and improved libido and mood.

Eat a diet that is balanced, refer to the alkaline dieting program.

Repeat/Reconnect

Always start your day meditating and visualizing the health, weight, and life goals and associate good feelings to them, remember, you are on your way to achieving them, when doubt enters your mind, flip switch it to the opposite positive affirmative thoughts.

Restore/Restart

We are creatures of habit. If you snap back to the old patterns, know that it's ok, just simply let it go and start over. Remember, insanity is doing the same things expecting different results. You are here to make a change, change your perception which will ultimately be your reality. The life of abundance, health, and happiness awaits you.

Section 3:
Basal Ganglia

The basal ganglia is the part of the brain that surrounds the deep limbic system. It is responsible for movement, thoughts, and feelings. When the basal ganglia are overactive, people tend to be immobile, and when it is under active, situations tend to trigger them to action. The two common dysfunctions with the basal ganglia are Parkinson's disease (PD) and Tourette's syndrome (TS). PD is caused by deficiency in dopamine and it is characterized by tremors, rigidity, loss of agility, facial expression, and slow movements. Giving these individuals L-Dopa significantly improves the condition. TS involves a combination of motor and vocal tics lasting more than a year.

Dysfunctions in the basal ganglia can lead to the following:

- anxiety/nervousness
- panic attacks
- negative outlook
- passive
- muscle tension
- tremors
- low/excessive motivation

The two neurotransmitters that are necessary in the brain are the serotonin and dopamine. There needs to be a right balance between the two neurotransmitters in the brain, this is tipped in the basal ganglia. Dopamine is involved with motor control, attention, motivation, and setting the motor speed. Serotonin is involved with mood control, shifting attention, and cognitive flexibility. The basal ganglia is involved with dopamine production.

Do you suspect you or anyone you know to have a dysfunction in the basal ganglia? Below are some symptoms.

- Nervousness/anxiety
- Panic Attacks
- Headaches

- Muscle tension

- Dizzy/faint

- Cold flash, cold hands

- Negative thoughts

- Passive

- Phobia

- Decreased/excessive motivation

- Tics

- Shy

- Poor handwriting

Healing the Basal Ganglia

The five R Matrix for the Basal Ganglia are as follows:

Recognize

Be aware of the triggers that cause you anxiety and write them down. Notice the autonomic thoughts that enter your mind and just notice them.

Remove

It takes some effort to alter your patterned thinking as they tend to be automatic. We have a tendency to generalize, delete, and distort all sensory information to what we believe. Therefore if what you believe is negative, then you have a tendency to generalize, delete, and distort the information to confirm your belief.

Just notice these negative tendencies and if they don't serve you and your life, switch the switch as you would a light switch from negative to positive. As long as you "notice" what happens in your processing the information, and find that it's not serving you, you will stop the pattern. Take a deep breath and tell yourself, "my perception is my reality, I create my life".

If conflicts arise in your life whether at work, home, or social, remember to detach yourself from the situation and remember that there is no meaning in anything until we place on there. Other people will always have their own opinions, don't let their opinions affect how you feel about yourself. When you speak, speak with conviction and mean what you say. Always maintain self control, this helps if you learn to detach yourself from a given situation, we usually infuse our personal emotional charge into a situation.

Replenish/Reprogram

Practice daily meditation, this helps to reset the basal ganglia to a calm level. The practice of meditation has many benefits proven by research including decreased anxiety, decreased blood pressure, and decreased stress. I recommend taking out the first 15-20 minutes a day in the morning to just sit quietly and imagine a place where you feel most at ease, is it a beach, mountain, whatever works for you and sense the smell, air, hear the surroundings, and taste what makes you feel at ease. The more detailed you can get about this special place, the better results that you can have. If and when your thoughts are swayed, just notice them but don't swell on them, take a long deep breath and just enjoy just "being" without any titles, identity, or responsibilities.

Choose to follow the alkaline dieting program which advise a balanced diet that keep you supplied with energy through the day. Remember, limit your intake of alcohol and caffeinated beverages, refined/processed foods, and sugar to a minimum. They can worsen your anxiety and fuel the wrong appetite, causing a vicious cycle. In my experience, this is why diets do not work because people tend to link emotions into eating and eating has become a habit.

Taking a bath (the ultimate half bath) as discussed in the alkaline abs is very helpful. I take regular baths in this salt solution to detoxify my body, mind, and soul. My patients have found it helpful to use essential oils in the water and/or use candles which have a calming effect.

Repeat/Reconnect

Always start your day meditating and visualizing the health, weight, and life goals and associate good feelings to them, remember, you are on your way to achieving them, when doubt enters your mind, flip switch it to the opposite positive affirmative thoughts.

Restore/Restart

We are creatures of habit. If you snap back to the old patterns, know that it's ok, just simply let it go and start over. Remember, insanity is doing the same things expecting different results. You are here to make a change, change your perception which will ultimately be your reality. The life of abundance, health, and happiness awaits you.

Section 4:
The Prefrontal Cortex

The prefrontal cortex (PFC) is the most evolved part of our brain. The PFC is responsible for higher level functions such as time management, critical thinking, impulse control, forward thinking, planning, and communication with others. It orchestrates the behavior.

PFC is the part of the brain there it allows you to be strategic in what and how you say or do prior to actually doing it. It guides you to problem solve, formulate goals, make plans, and execute them. This part of the brain also allows you insight to learn from your mistakes from your past.

The PFC also responsible for having sustained focus or attention. It allows you to take in important information through the filtering process. This area of the brain communicates with the primitive part of the brain, both the basal ganglia and the limbic system. The PFC interprets the sensory input into feelings and emotions and allows for proper expression with words to convey love, passion, and dislike. The PFC shares many inputs and outputs into the limbic system, sending inhibitory signals to refrain from certain activities. When there is a dysfunction with the PFC, the following may manifest:

- Lack of focus
- Lack of impulse control
- Hyperactive behavior
- Lack or order
- Lack of emotion
- Poor judgment
- Anxiety
- Poor time management
- Decreased information processing "slow" to respond
- Lack of behavioral control
- Moodiness

Do you suspect that you or anyone you know have PFC dysfunction?

- Difficulty with sustained attention

- Constantly makes careless mistakes

- Difficulty with expressing emotions, empathy or sympathy

- Lack of time management

- Lack of follow through and finishing tasks

- Blurt out answers before the question is asked

- Trouble sitting still

- Easily bored

- Excessive day dream

- Lack of motivation

- Lethargic

- Lacking social etiquette (impulsive social interaction)

- Make repetitive mistakes that one's made in the past

Become focused prescription

The five R matrix:

<u>Recognize</u>

Awareness of your tendencies is first and foremost before you are able to accept responsibility and make necessary changes. Just observe your behaviors and how it manifests, just notice what you do in a given situation. See also if there are triggers that exacerbate the PFC dysfunction.

Sometimes, taking the time to journal these events are helpful to allow you to really reflect on your behavior and to make necessary adjustments.

<u>Remove</u>

Eliminate any triggers, situations that disrupt focus as the prefrontal cortex is responsible for focus, attention, and concentration. This trigger can be in the form of people, objects, noise, etc. Just remove them altogether and notice how you are able to focus.

Since PFC dysfunctional individuals tend to be conflict seeking for increased stimulation, avoid feeding the internal conflict and take deep breaths until the urge to argue subsides.

Replenish/Reprogram

Add meaning, purpose, and stimulation to your life for added excitement, your prefrontal cortex needs it to excel. For example, people with ADD (attention deficit disorder) often struggle with mundane and boring day to day routines. On the other hand, they excel when there is a challenge that stimulates the PFC.

Organization and order is important for the PFC to heal. Typically, PFC dysfunctions can cause problems with organization, learning to organize and plan is very helpful.

- Keep a pocket calendar
- Keep a "To Do" list
- Prioritize your responsibilities
- Break down the bigger projects that overwhelm you
- Keep deadlines
- Consider hiring a professional organizer

Pay also special attention to the diet. A diet that is balanced will deliver steady level of energy. Avoid refined and processed foods that are high in additives and artificial compounds, rather choose whole fruits and vegetables that are in season. Avoid alcohol and soda. Refer to the alkaline dieting program for details on how to eat for optimal health and concentration.

Repeat/Reconnect

It is human nature to snap back to our own selves. Don't be disappointed if and when you do make the same mistakes and your PFC dysfunctions dominate at times. Remember, consistency in our efforts will pay off. The neural connections are being formed, of course your old connections are more dominant as you've had more time to program them. Give yourself a break and understand that the new ones are being formed and so keep going, just keep doing.

Restore/Restart

We are creatures of habit. If you snap back to the old patterns, know that it's ok, just simply let it go and start over. Remember, insanity is doing the same things expecting different results. You are here to make a change, change your perception which will ultimately be your reality.   The life of abundance, health, and happiness awaits you.

Section 5:
The Cingulate System

The cingulate gyrus runs longitudinal through the frontal lobes of the brain. This part of the brain allows you to shift your attention from one situation to another, one idea from another, and to have a healthy perspective of life. It is responsible for information processing and flexibility in its interpretation, cognitive flexibility as defined by Dr. Amen "Change your Brain, Change your life".

The cognitive flexibility allows for change and adaptation to new situations, processing new problems and coming up with solutions. Since life is constantly evolving with new situations and circumstances this flexibility is necessary for one to thrive. The cingulate system is also involved with planning and goal setting.

Let's now consider the dysfunctions in the cingulate system, an individual with cingulate dysfunction may exhibit the following:

- Excessive worrying

- Holding on to the problems and scars of the past

- Getting stuck on thoughts

- Argumentative

- Lack of cooperation

- Addictive behaviors

- Difficulty with adapting to new situations

- Compulsive behaviors

- Eating Disorders

- Anger issues

- Obsessive Compulsive Disorders

Individuals with the dysfunctions in the cingulate system have tendencies to dwell and get stuck on issues by rethinking the thought repeatedly. They tend to hold grudges from the past, allowing it to run their lives even though its toxic to their future. On the OCD spectrum, they may wash hands over and over, excessively checking to see if they locked the door, etc.

These individuals can be difficult to deal with because they are incapable of shifting thoughts, for example, they only know one way of doing things such as putting away the dishes a specific way, avoid love making because the bed might be messy after, or insisting on eating one kind of food and avoiding different foods without any consideration. The most difficult is the automatic "no" attitude. I had a business partner in the past where every new idea that I would recommend that we try, he would tell me numerous reasons why it could not be done. He was incapable of finding out the solutions to make it happen, rather he was "stuck" in the fact that it could not be done without any factual evidence to support this. Needless to say, our partnership ended.

I also have two sons; the younger son on occasion demonstrates this behavior. On a hot summer day, he would insist on wearing his winter spider man snow boots. I've tried every different reasoning to insist that it's ludicrous for him to wear this boot to no avail on many occasions. I found that redirecting his attention to something else such as focusing on a different topic, like going for ice cream, which flavor he would like, would allow him to shift and forget about the boot issue. It can be frustrating to deal with at times, but if we understand that it's a physiological issue that they can't help, it's helpful to find a solution to get along.

Do you or anyone you know have overactive cingulate system?

- Excessive worrying
- Obsessive cleaning
- Excessive attachment to their habit
- Reluctance to change
- Anger outrage
- Tendency for addictive behaviors (alcohol, gambling, eating disorders, smoking, etc.)
- Difficulty changing perspective
- Tendency to expect the negative outcome

• Demanding to do things their way.

Let's talk about dealing with the individuals with the cingulate dysfunctions. It is important to note that changing behaviors can alter brain wave patterns by way of the neural synaptic changes as discussed in the earlier sections.

Recognize

Notice when you get stuck and simply distract yourself with other thoughts and come back to the issue later. This gives your brain a break and allows for more adaptability. For example, my brother had a tendency to worry excessively and complained that he can't break from this thought. He was studying for the boards for chiropractic exam and was thinking that he could not pass despite all his efforts in preparing for the test. I advised him to think about the bible verse that he likes and repeat it in his mind twenty times when this occurs. He told me that this had allowed him to overcome his constant worrying, not only was he able to pass the boards, but he's got a number of bible verses memorized.

Remove

When unrelenting anger, compulsion for a certain behavior, or when you are stuck dealing with an individual who are also "stuck", remove yourself from the situation, if physical removal is not possible then a mental removal works just fine. Just repeat a favorite verse of any kind for a minute, take long slow breaths, and deal with the situation at a later time. You will find that this technique will prevent you from making mistakes that you'll regret and keep you from frustrations.

My favorite go to verse in the bible is:

John 16:33 I have said these things to you, that in me you may have peace. In the world you will have tribulation. But take heart; I have overcome the world."

Replenish/Reprogram

I'm sure you've heard of the term "reverse psychology". With cingulate individuals, this technique works. Ask the opposite of what you want. I used this with my younger son; he was once on a rampage about how much he hated me because I repositioned his toy from one place to another. I asked him for a hug shortly after that after apologizing and he downright refused. Then I said, please don't give me a hug because I don't want one from an angry boy and he readily came and could not keep himself from me telling me how much he loved me.

Sometimes, seeking wise counsel will help you deal with the situation. I believe having a good mentor or a confidante that you can trust and who supports you can provide a good sounding board for you. This allows you to build a good foundation and understand your behaviors so that you can alter and change your perceptions to get better outcome, which will help you to succeed in life. Doing these steps, recognizing, removing, and then replenishing to reprogram your mind prior to you acting out of impulses will allow you more flexibility and also permit your brain to adapt to this new behavior by making new neural connections for growth and change for an optimal outcome.

Repeat/Reconnect

Remember not to get disappointed if you revert back sometimes. Our programming is strong, it took the amount of time to be programmed into us, it's not going to be as easy as a click of a button. However, remember, that the neural connections are being made and it takes approximately 21-30 days for a habit to become ingrained in us. Key thing is to keep doing, your efforts will pay off, I promise, before you know it, you won't remember the last time you were worried, angry, or obsessive. Your problems will seem so small and your outlook so bright.

Restore/Restart

We are creatures of habit. If you snap back to the old patterns, know that it's ok, just simply let it go and start over. Remember, insanity is doing the same things expecting different results. You are here to make a change, change your perception which will ultimately be your reality. The life of abundance, health, and happiness awaits you.

Section 6:
Temporal Lobes

The functions of the temporal lobes are the most important in my opinion. The temporal lobes allow you to:

- Process and understand language

- Have memory

- Enable auditory learning

- Allow for emotional stability

- Recognize facial expressions

- Enable visual learning

- Music appreciation

- Define who we are

Temporal lobes are divided into two sides, the left and right. Depending on which side your dominant side is, the processing may vary. For example, the left lobe (dominant side for most), is responsible for processing language, memory storage, emotional stability, and visual and auditory processing.

Language allows for communication with each other, exchanging ideas and self-expression of our thoughts and actions. It is also the hallmark of being human.

The right lobe (the non-dominant for most) is involved with reading facial expressions, processing verbal tones, music appreciation, and visual learning. The ability to recognize faces, interpret intonations of the voices set the foundation for healthy social skills. Being able to know when someone is scared of you, happy to see you, or not interested in you is key for interpersonal connection.

Let's then explore the problems that one can have with temporal lobe dysfunction.

- Excess aggression

- Mild paranoia

- Difficulty with word retrieval

- Difficulty with reading

- Emotional instability

- Difficulty with memory recall

- Anxiety for no reason

- Confusion

- Social struggles

- Difficulty with facial recognition

- Seizures

- Illusions

Reflecting on the people around you, I'm sure you know someone that may have temporal lobe dysfunctions. It's important to note that the issues may be falsely categorized as psychotic when it is purely biological in nature. Due to the anatomical place of the temporal lobe, it sits behind sharp bony ridge which can be frequently damaged with the slight trauma to the head.

Remember that the temporal lobes allow for defining the essence of who you are. It also houses the memory and can directly affect our outlook on life.

Let's now discuss the five R matrix for the temporal lobe dysfunction:

Recognize

Notice your behavior and see if any of the list of dysfunctions apply to you or someone you know. Recognizing and correctly understanding the underlying reason is very important for correct diagnosis and finding solutions to be more effective and happy.

Remove

If you have had a traumatic life event, and recognize that this event is negatively affecting the choices you make and give emotional instability, take deep breaths when this occurs. Here is a technique that I want you to try; it's been very effective for me.

Just notice the event and recall the event as you stay far away from your own body as the event is being recalled. Just welcome any negative emotions that it brings up and just notice them and embrace them. Then, just let it go far away from you as if you are freeing yourself from the burden of this event and all its effects in your life. You see, we often carry the negative event and it becomes the very fiber of our being. We become cingulate in our thinking and have a tendency to want to hold on to this negative event deep within us. Just let it go.........detach from it. See yourself, do this from far away and let it go without attaching any meaning. Understand that we create our reality; there is no inherent meaning in anything, any events, or any comments from others until we ourselves place them there. This technique allows you to detach from your hurtful past. I've had to do this myself and has really transformed my marriage and my family life.

Avoid caffeine, nicotine, and alcohol. The caffeine and nicotine are strong vasoconstrictors that decrease blood flow and nutrition to the brain.

Replenish/Reprogram

Keeping your temporal lobe stimulated with positive memories will keep you excited and joyfully motivated. Make your experiences count by enjoying every day and celebrating life. Keep count of all the special and joyful memories and replay them as you wish. If you have difficulty with them, then create your own memory by visualization technique. Think of what you want, how you would like to live, how you would like you relationships and then just create a movie of it in your mind and play them daily. It is scientifically proven that the thoughts have energy and that it can play an important role in your energy level.

Sing on a regular basis, as a Christian, I sing and listen to the hymnals on a regular basis which allows me to be in a bright mood centered in my faith. Meditate for about 10 minutes to start and working up to 30 minutes or more. This really allows your mind to reset and recharge from all the "noise" of our mind. Breath consciously, inhale and exhale without a break and just notice your body, how it just knows when to breath in and out. The wonders of our body is representation of the higher God. By doing this, you are allowing the neural connections to take a break and rest.

Get enough sleep. It is idea to have between 6-8 hours a sleep a night for optimal performance. Sleep is associated with improved mood, focus, emotional stability, and improved cognitive ability.

Let's not forget to mention the importance of proper nutrition. Consume plenty of fruits and vegetables, fish, and whole grains. It is important to note to decrease intake of refined and processed foods that are high in sugar. Sugar exacerbates the temporal lobe dysfunctions and can increase irritability, and aggressive behaviors.

Repeat/Reconnect

Once you understand the inner workings of your mind, keep the cycle going on different behaviors by repeating the same process over again. Remember, it takes 21-30 days for habits to sink it, until then, it's not so autonomic. It takes repeated practices, keep your focus on the goal.

Restore/Restart

It may take multiple run throughs to really grasp any given behavior, your brain has a learning curve. If you happen to fall off track just get right back and restart the cycle all over again to ensure that you will continue to get the ultimate outcome that you desire.

Section 7:
Stress

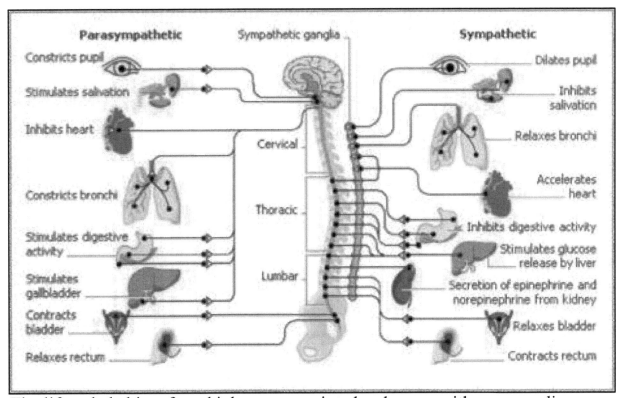

The lifestyle habits of our high strung society burdens us with never ending stress. Stress of economic melt downs, stress of raising kids in this highly technical world, the stress of aging parents, stress of holding onto jobs, and stress of work life balance is on the rise. Everywhere you look it seems that everyone is bombarded with too much to do, not enough time. This is why the health of America is declining with so many convenient options for foods from microwave dinners to drive through meals. We are eating on the run, it's harder and harder to maintain the family unity as the dinners are replaced with drive through on the way to soccer practice, grab on the go for executives, its common to see individuals eating while driving, eating is no longer a sacred ritual. It's all about how much you can fit in a given day. Even when you do get the family together, it is common place to see families all entertaining themselves with smart phones rather than having healthy conversations and bonding with each other. Let us first define stress.

The term "stress", as it is currently used was coined by Hans Selye in 1936, who defined it as "the non-specific response of the body to any demand for change". Selye had noted in numerous experiments that laboratory animals subjected to acute but different noxious physical and emotional stimuli (blaring light, deafening noise, extremes of heat or cold, perpetual frustration) all exhibited the same pathologic changes of stomach ulcerations, shrinkage of lymphoid tissue and enlargement of the adrenals. He later demonstrated that persistent stress could cause these animals to develop various diseases similar to those seen in humans, such as heart attacks, stroke, kidney disease and rheumatoid arthritis. At the time, it was believed that most diseases were caused by specific but different pathogens. Tuberculosis was due to the tubercle bacillus, anthrax by the anthrax bacillus, syphilis by a spirochete, etc. What Selye proposed was just the opposite, namely that many different insults could cause the same disease, not only in animals, but in humans as well. (American Institute of Stress)

Selye's theories popularized the use of the word stress. Until recently, the word stress was completely foreign to me. As a western trained clinician and a patient, whenever I heard the disease was caused by "stress" I dismissed this theory as being woo woo. I needed objective answers to my problems both with my diagnosis of Lupus and when treating patients.

Because it was apparent that most people viewed stress as some unpleasant threat, Selye subsequently had to create a new word, stressor, to distinguish stimulus from response. Stress was generally considered as being synonymous with distress and dictionaries defined it as "physical, mental, or emotional strain or tension" or "a condition or feeling experienced when a person perceives that demands exceed the personal and social resources the individual is able to mobilize." Thus, stress was put in a negative light and its positive effects ignored. However, stress can be helpful and good when it motivates people to accomplish more. (American Institute of Stress)

Selye struggled unsuccessfully all his life to find a satisfactory definition of stress. In attempting to extrapolate his animal studies to humans so that people would understand what he meant, he redefined stress as "The rate of wear and tear on the body". This is actually a pretty good description of biological aging so it is not surprising that increased stress can accelerate many aspects of the aging process. In his later years, when asked to define stress, he told reporters, "Everyone knows what stress is, but nobody really knows."

As noted, stress is difficult to define because it is so different for each of us. A good example is afforded by observing passengers on a steep roller coaster ride. Some are hunched down in the back seats, eyes shut, jaws clenched and white knuckled with an iron grip on the retaining bar. They can't wait for the ride in the torture chamber to end so they can get back on solid ground and scamper away. But up front are the wide-eyed thrill seekers, yelling and relishing each steep plunge who race to get on the very next ride. And in between you may find a few with an air of nonchalance that borders on boredom. So, was the roller coaster ride stressful? (American Institute of Stress)

As with the roller coaster analogy, the same stressor can affect us differently. It is our individual perceptions of the stressor that dictate the impact on us physically. There are plenty of research to prove that increased stress can directly impact the physiology of our systemic functions which can alter immune system, cardio-metabolic system, the endocrine system, the nervous system, the digestive system, and the hormonal system.

Clinically we know that stress can manifest into physiological symptoms including fatigue, irritable bowel syndrome, acid reflux, fatigue, autoimmune disease, diabetes, high blood pressure, etc.

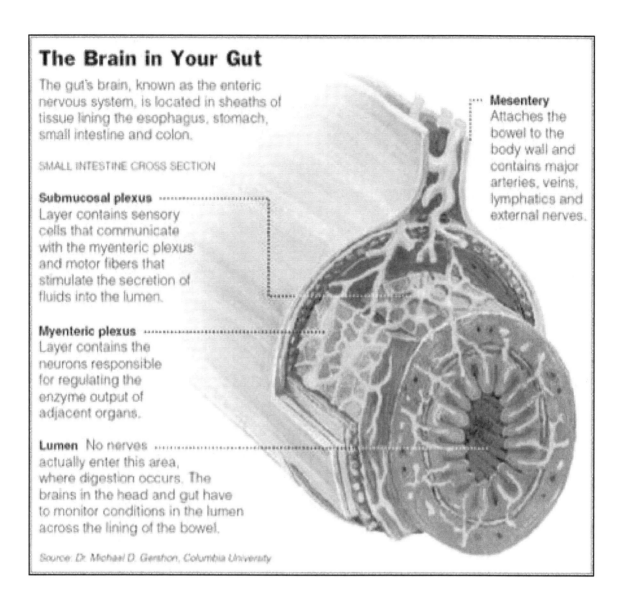

The Brain in Your Gut

The gut's brain, known as the enteric nervous system, is located in sheaths of tissue lining the esophagus, stomach, small intestine and colon.

SMALL INTESTINE CROSS SECTION

Submucosal plexus
Layer contains sensory cells that communicate with the myenteric plexus and motor fibers that stimulate the secretion of fluids into the lumen.

Myenteric plexus
Layer contains the neurons responsible for regulating the enzyme output of adjacent organs.

Lumen No nerves actually enter this area, where digestion occurs. The brains in the head and gut have to monitor conditions in the lumen across the lining of the bowel.

Source: Dr. Michael D. Gershon, Columbia University

Mesentery
Attaches the bowel to the body wall and contains major arteries, veins, lymphatics and external nerves.

Stress cascade can alter and modulate the hormonal secretions of the endocrine system, the digestive abilities can be negatively altered and mutate the cellular divisions and genes and create a tumor within our bodies that can potentially lead to cancer. This cascade also can affect the body by lowering the threshold of the disease and turn on the silent disease genes and create numerous antibodies to give rise to various autoimmune diseases. Deepak Chopra has long been talking about psychoneuroimmunology and he talks extensively about the condition of the mind to trigger various neurotransmitters and neural connections that allow for disease onset via altering various organs through its neurochemical alterations that can affect a change in the cascade which can ultimately lead to genetic mutations which can lead to various medical conditions. The primary system that this can impact is the digestive system. In eastern medicine as well as in functional medicine, they look to the digestive process as the culprit to all diseases. This is where the environment can be assimilated via food. Obviously, if the food contains toxins and foreign substance that the human body cannot completely digest with ease, it can start the inflammatory cascade and alter the gut flora and immune response activated. Refer to the image.

How then does one cope with stress?

I am sure you or someone you know suffers from increased stress. The most important factor into taking a hold of stress is to notice what they are. Then take charge and take control of the stress rather than letting it take control of you.

When I was running three different businesses and raising two toddlers, my days were never long enough. Although I always knew that I needed to take it easy, I never really can gauge how much stress I was taking on. It is very difficult to measure. For me, I began to have lupus flares, unexplained rashes, extreme fatigue, depression, anxiety, and nervous breakdowns. The thing was even though I was extremely tired, I was too wired with "to do" lists to sleep. I really needed to slow down. Through trial and error, it helped me tremendously to learn more about me and my stressors by examining and taking the five R Matrix implementation. My life is very different today. I no longer have stress not because I don't have any but because I nip it in the bud before it can affect me. Take the five Matrix system to defeat your own stress before it takes over your life.

Recognize

Take a survey of your life. It is helpful to write down the very things that you think about daily. Once you jot this down you will find that most of your stressors are in front of you. Then, take a few days and just notice what you do whenever the certain stressor is mentioned, do you avoid it, do you get depressed, does your heart beat faster, do you start to eat? Just notice the physiological and emotional response to the stressors. My stressors are the book that I am writing, cooking for my family, my family relationships, my health, my business, etc.

Remove

Once you are clear about your stressors, one by one as they come up, alter your response by writing down what the worst situation of this stressor can bring. Often times than not, you will find that whatever you are worried about does not have any rhyme or reason to worry you at all. In other words, you are "conditioned" to worry and it's almost an autonomic response for you.

Remember the part of the brain that is responsible for worrying? Yes, the cingulate system. We have tendencies to hold on to the negatives in our lives, we let them in to the very fibers of our being. It may be a negative experience that may consume you to over worry but really when you take the time to survey and reflect on what it is that you are worried about, almost always, it does not warrant this amount of energy.

Like a light switch, turn off the negative thought and flip switch to the positive.

Replenish/Reprogram

Once you have begun the positive thinking process, close your eyes and visualize the positive outcome. If it's a boss at work who stresses you out, just visualize her/him being nice to you and complimenting your work rather than reprimanding. If it's the deadline that you have to meet, instead of thinking that you can't meet it, visualize that you have already met the deadline and enjoying the glass of wine. Remember, the new neural connection that we are making takes some time to be automatic. Keep doing this flip switching from negative to positive, I promise you'll get the result that you want of having the best life that you've ever wanted.

Repeat/Reconnect

This takes practice; don't get discouraged if after a few good weeks you fall back into your own patterned behavior. You will find that the pull of your will to revert back is ever so strong because you ego knows nothing more than what you have programmed. Once you keep doing this, this pull to the old you will diminish and your desired attitude will be automatic. Whenever I implement the five R matrix to any areas of my life, I fight the ego battle by visualizing the desired outcome rather than feeding my mind fear of not accomplishing it. Remember, where your mind goes, your attention goes, your energy works in this direction to create the desired outcome. On the flip side, if you constantly think of what you are trying to avoid, what if's , then your mind will be the faithful servant by getting you the very thing that you don't simply because that is what you are thinking. You avoiding the negative outcome should be replaced with what would happen if all goes well...

Restore/Restart

In no time at all, you will notice that you are changing, not a temporary transient willed change, but you will find that you create your life and do things that serve you effortlessly. You'll find that you too can create magic.

On the next section, you will find a questionnaire that will help you to quantify stress. Take it for fun and see how much stress you are living with. The higher the total score, the higher level of stress that you have. The test is compliments of Metagenics.

Section 8:
Stress Assessment

Identi- T TM Stress Assessment

Name_____

Age _____

Sex _____

Date_____

Stress is a normal part of life. Every day, we're faced with stimuli, called stressors, which can elicit the body's "fight or flight" response, setting off a cascade of physiological reactions and resulting in emotions ranging from mild to intense. But while occasional stress is natural and even healthy, chronic or acute stress can be harmful.

Please take a few moments to discover your body's response to situations you perceive as stressful. By honestly assessing how you feel, your healthcare provider can create a natural stress relief program for your individual needs.

Directions:

Please read each statement and circle the number 0, 1, 2, or 3 that best describes your feelings or reactions throughout the course of the day. Determine the subtotal score for each section, then determine the total scores for sections A-C and C-E. Some questions may appear redundant between sections. There's a reason for each question. Don't spend much time on any one question.

0 = Never true 1= Seldom true 2= Sometimes true 3= Often true

For the last two weeks or longer, I...

Section A:

1.   Get wound up when I get tired and have trouble calming down   0   1   2   3

2.   Feel driven, appear energetic but feel "burned out" and exhausted
      0   1   2   3

3.   Feel restless, agitated, anxious, and uneasy

      0   1   2   3

6. Feel easily overwhelmed by emotion. 0   1   2   3

7. Feel emotional — cry easily or laugh inappropriately.   0   1   2   3

8. Experience heart palpitations or a pounding in my chest

      0   1   2   3

9. I am short of breath   0   1   2   3

8. Am constipated   0   1   2   3

10. Feel warm, over-heated, and dry all over   0   1   2   3

11. Get mouth sores or sore tongue 0   1   2   3

12. Get hot flashes 0   1   2   3

13. Sleep less than seven hours a night   0   1   2   3

14. Have trouble falling asleep and staying asleep

      0   1   2   3

15. Worry about high blood pressure, cholesterol, and triglycerides 0   1   2   3

16. Forget to eat and feel little hunger   0   1   2   3

Section B:

17. Find myself worrying about things big and small

      0   1   2   3

18. Feel like I can't stop worrying, even though I want to

      0   1   2   3

19. Feel impulsive, pent up, and ready to explode

      0   1   2   3

20. Get muscle spasms 0   1   2   3

21. Feel aggressive, unyielding, or inflexible when pressed for time   0   1   2   3

22. See, hear, and smell things that others do not

    0   1   2   3

23. Stay awake replaying the events of the day or planning for tomorrow   0   1   2   3

24. Have upsetting thoughts or images enter my mind again and again   0   1   2   3

25. Have a hard time stopping myself from doing things again and again, like checking on things or rearranging objects over and over   0   1   2   3

26. Worry a lot about terrible things that could happen if I'm not careful   0   1   2   3

Section C:

27. Have muscle and joint pains.   0   1   2   3

28. Have muscle weakness   0   1   2   3

29. Crave salt or salty things 0   1   2   3

30. Have multiple points on my body that when touched are tender or painful   0   1   2   3

31. Have dark circles under my eyes 0   1   2   3

32. Feel a sudden sense of anxiety when I get hungry

    0   1   2   3

33. Use medications to manage pain   0   1   2   3

34. Get dizzy when rising or standing up from a kneeling or sitting position   0   1   2   3

35. Have diarrhea or bouts of nausea with or without vomiting for no apparent reason   0   1   2   3

36. Have headaches   0   1   2   3

Total points: _____

Section D:

1. Have trouble organizing my thoughts   0   1   2   3

2. Get easily distracted and lose focus

37. Have difficulty making decisions and mistrust my judgment   0   1   2   3

38. Feel depressed and apathetic   0   1   2   3

39. Lack the motivation and energy to stay on task and pay attention   0   1   2   3

40. Am forgetful   0   1   2   3

41. Feel unsettled, restless, and anxious   0   1   2   3

42. Wake up tired and unrefreshed   0   1   2   3

43. Experience heartburn and indigestion   0   1   2   3

44. Catch colds or infections easily   0   1   2   3

Total points:

Section E:

45. Feel tired for no apparent reason.   0   1   2   3

46. Experience lingering mild fatigue after exertion or physical activity   0   1   2   3

47. Find it difficult to concentrate and complete tasks

        0   1   2   3

48. Feel depressed and apathetic   0   1   2   3

49. Feel cold or chilled – hands, feet, or all over – for no apparent reason   0   1   2   3

50. Have little or no interest in sex   0   1   2   3

51. Sweat spontaneously during the day   0   1   2   3

52. Feel puffy and retain fluids   0   1   2   3

53. Sleep more than nine hours a night   0   1   2   3

54. Have poor muscle tone 0 1 2 3

55. Have trouble losing weight 0 1 2 3

56. Wake up tired even though I seem to get plenty of sleep

 0 1 2 3

57. Have no energy and feel physically weak 0 1 2 3

58. Am susceptible to colds and the flu 0 1 2 3

59. Feel dragged down by multiple symptoms, such as poor digestion and body aches 0 1 2 3

Add points from sections A, B & C

Total for A, B & C: _____

Add points from sections C, D & E

Total for C, D & E: _____

Lifestyle and Health Status:

60. Circle the level of stress you experience on the scale of 1-10, 10 being the worst: 1 2 3 4 5 6 7 8 9 10

61. What do you consider to be the major causes of your stress (for example — spouse, family, friends, work, finances, wedding, pregnancy,

62. legal, commute):

_____

_____

_____

___

63. I eat breakfast _____ times a week. My typical breakfast is:

_____

_____

_____

64. I take a multiple vitamin/mineral _____ days per week. I take a fish oil supplement _____ days per week.

65. I participate in 30 minutes of physical activity such as walking, aerobics (e.g., running), resistance training (e.g., weights, pilates), sports (e.g. biking), or yoga:

66. Daily _____ 5-6 times per week_____ 3-4 times per week_____ 1-2 times per week_____

    Less than once a week _____

    a. I smoke _____ cigarettes daily. I drink two or more 8 ounce cups of caffeinated coffee or other caffeinated beverages like energy/diet drinks, colas, or black or green teas:

    b. Daily_____ 5-6 times per week_____

       3-4 times per week_____ 1-2 times per week _____

       Less than once a week _____

67. I drink two or more ounces of alcoholic beverages:

68. Daily _____ 5-6 times per week_____

    3-4 times per week_____ 1-2 times per week_____ Less than once a week _____

69. List your current health problems and any over-the-counter or prescription medications that you are now taking:

    _____

    _____

    _____

Section 9:
What's your mind got to do with it?

As a person with chronic disease, my personal mission for my life is to allow my body to heal and help others to do the same.

All my years of didactic and formal training has taught me to look to the hard core evidence in all things that are proven scientific. Most of you are aware that I am constantly striving to gain more knowledge. I am committed to further my education mainly because I feel that my questions have not been answered.

For the last 12 years, oriental medicine, or TCM (traditional Chinese Medicine) was under my radar, just never pursued due to not enough scientific research to validate the findings, or so I thought. As I researched and read deeper, I've come to conclude that the state of our health has everything to do with our thoughts.

Medical research is finding that the nature of our thoughts and actions determine our physical structure and function of our bodies. This has its strong evidence in the case of the "placebo" effect. The placebo effect is when the mind is tested into thinking that they are given a medical intervention for the symptoms when in reality they weren't given anything. They found that the placebo effect has better or same effect as the actual drug in a group of subjects. It is safe to conclude that this is because the mind was deceived into believing that they were given an intervention. Take a moment and think about the implications of this.......your thoughts can dictate the health of your body.

Can your mind control your health status? Yes. Universe is a master piece of abundance and health. Good health, wealth, nature.....negative thoughts cut you off from the natural resources of well being. Have you heard of the term, being in the same frequency with someone? I'm sure all of you experienced being around someone with negative attitude....it really can dampen your mood, have you wondered why? It's because our attitudes control our physiological vibrations which create a frequency. The vibrational energy creates an aura around you and emits a frequency into the universe. This may sound voodoo, but it's all proven quantum physics.

Dis- ease body is not at ease.....Disease is result of stress. You put enough stress in the body and one of the links break. This is the threshold of your health, disease manifests when the body reaches a threshold, which is different for everyone. The good news is that with the power of right thinking, you can heal. Laughter is the medicine, food is medicine, you have a body that is innately programmed to heal and be healthy.

Remember that the disease cannot live in a body that is at a positive frequency. We reproduce everyday at the cellular level, which means that within a few years, we have a new body.

Take home message, visualize yourself with perfect health. You choose to live in joy or choose to live in sorrow, knowing what you know about the power of the mind, why would you live in the latter. Don't focus on what's wrong, because you'll only perpetuate it, focus on the good things in life and be grateful for them. Happier thoughts = happier biochemistry = Healthy body= Life of abundance

Remember, Incurable is curable from within.

I am thankful for everyday and want to live a live that is fulfilling, that is to serve you.

Part II:
Alkaline Abs

"An early-morning walk is a blessing for the whole day."
— *Henry David Thoreau*

The alkaline program is a comprehensive program addressing the whole body, mind and spirit to provide you with the tools for transformative changes that will have you locked in the life of abundance, health, and happiness.

My background in exercise and movement started with Jane Fonda workouts back 24 years ago. As a teenager trying to look the part and also one wanting to maintain the weight, I remember following Jane Fonda VHS cassettes from my own living room. I was a dancer and believed the cardiovascular benefit will serve me well.....I was thinking, "this should tone me up".

As I matured, I sought various forms of exercise and tried everything from kick-boxing, aerobics, step aerobics, sculpting classes, elliptical, and running. I was introduced to yoga during my graduate study in nutrition. Due to limited access to classes at the local gym, I found a yoga DVD of Kathy Smith and I began to practice daily. I liked the practice, I felt it grounded me and revived my whole body. It wasn't easy in the beginning, however, as I improved, I liked it more and more. However, I was only interested in the physical outer benefit of long, lean, and toned body. As a Christian, my obstacle was to demystify the belief that yoga is another form of religion, that it was rooted in Hinduism, something to stay away from. Now I know that it's far from the truth.

With the onset of my Lupus diagnosis, I began to have much joint and muscle pain. I sought alternative exercises, practiced much advanced yoga DVD's and the VHS tapes as the yoga classes were not conducted at a local gym at that time. Then, my natural inclination of performing more resistive exercises began to surface and found that Pilates provided just that. As my body was weaker with intake of harmful medications such as corticosteroids, my muscles were shrinking and I felt very weak.

Since I was a doctoral student in physical therapy, I felt I wanted to pursue some form of certification that will enhance my profession. I researched the Los Angeles area for a Pilates Training facility. Pilates over yoga because I felt Pilates resonated and was more in line with the physical therapy practice. I found a colleague in Santa Monica, however, my schedule did not permit the training which required ample time both in practice and as an apprentice.

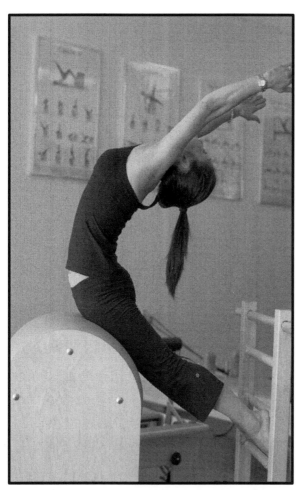

Fast forward 5 years and my son was 15 months, I had a severe relapse in Lupus which resulted in high doses of corticosteroid and chemotherapy. I was severely weak and knew at the time that I needed to stay healthy and strong for my baby. More than anything, I did not like the physical effects of rounded face, weight gain, and racing heart beat. I decided to start the comprehensive training in Pilates with the vision of helping other women like me by opening a wellness center in my neighborhood.

I also went for training in therapeutic yoga because I knew that there was a place for both. I spent the last 8 years perfecting the practice and learning the similarities and differences between yoga and pilates. I learned that there is political opposition between different schools of teachings from Traditional Pilates to Conventional, Deep practice of traditional Indian culture infused yoga to the watered down studios emerging throughout the world. I reviewed and researched all aspects. I knew there had to be a better way, to simplify the benefits of the practices and bring them to you. During my journey, I came across the traditional Asian rooted Qi Gong and Tai Chi. This too resonated with me as my spiritual journey of connecting to my true self was deepening and opening doors for me. I wanted nothing more than to just understand the way.

I began to compile all the knowledge I've gained and realized that all the practices have its place and the health benefits were profound. With my physical therapy, nutritional, and psychology background, I began to put together the comprehensive system that will transcend and complete each one of you to find your own internal thermostats and most importantly reset them.

The Alkaline Program will peel away all myths and complications and simplify the information in a way that you can digest, understand, and most importantly put into practice. Whether you are trying to heal from a disease, find true inner peace, or simply to lose weight, you will find that all paths lead to your ultimate goal and much more. Our lives and bodies are not a part of something, its the sum total of all its parts, mind, body, and spirit.

The Alkaline Program consists of three parts, the alkaline mind, alkaline abs (movement), and the alkaline dieting. While each program is complete on its own, it is important to note that the three parts work together to complete the program.

Alkaline Abs

As the section is about Alkaline Abs, it is important to note that there are two types of acidity, respiratory acidity and metabolic acidity. As the terms imply, the respiratory alkalinity involves breathing and CO_2 and possible accumulation of the lactic acid due to too much exercise. The metabolic acidity involves the diet and the metabolic acids that are formed due to poor food choices. For the purpose of the Alkaline Abs, we will focus on the respiratory pH. You will learn about the metabolic acidity in the Alkaline Dieting program.

1. Respiration/Breathing

Respiration/breathing is something that most of us don't think about, we are not aware of our breathing pattern or the way we breath. In the process of respiration, O_2 is breathed in and CO_2 is released. With the aerobic exercises for a prolonged periods or at a high intensity there is an increase in lactic acid as a byproduct which can decrease the pH, which is acidic.

It is important to know that exercise or movement is important in maintaining the health of our bodies. However, there are proper exercises that will keep our body in a healthy pH range. Follow the following and you will tone, dissolve belly fat, feel younger and have more vitality.

2. Postural Awareness.

As a physical therapist, this is the first thing I address no matter what the reason is for their seeking care. If you have bad posture, you are more prone to have blockages in energy flow to the head and the rest of the body and you can be sure that the health will decline as well. The shoulders should be back, standing tall, and abdominals engaged sot hold up the spine. Also if you keep your wallet in the back pocket of your pants (men), I would change to the front pockets because when you sit, you are creating an imbalance between your sit bones that can cause postural compensation that will affect the alignment of your spine, especially when sitting. Remember, the Modern American Lifestyle involves a lot of sitting in front of the computer, this is a long time to cause a dysfunctional posture through your day.

3. Mindful Breathing

As mentioned above, the respiration has an impact on the pH. I recommend that you breath with awareness allowing the rib cage to expand and extend the spine slightly with inhalation and contract and engage the abdominals as you exhale allowing the energy to flow through getting rid of all the CO_2 and breathing in the O_2. Before you can fully engage in proper breathing, you need to have an open posture so review above and make sure that you understand proper posture.

4. Exercise on a regular basis

Its important to be aware that too much of a good thing can be harmful. This is true in high intensity exercise due to increase lactic acid. I'm sure you've all be sore the day after a high intensity workout or after a strenuous weekend workout that we occasionally engage in, the term is a weekend warrior. This is thanks to the lactic acid in the muscles.

There are two types of exercises: Aerobic or Anaerobic, or Passive

I recommend the following for aerobic exercises:

Rebounding, walking, elliptical, or recumbent bike

I recommend the following for anaerobic which is great for stress relief, posture, toning, and flat abs...

Pilates, Yoga, Tai Chi, Qi Gong, my very own complete movement method, YoQiLates.

Passive is

Meditation

There is growing body of medical research validating the benefits of mediation, this is again due to our MAL (modern American Lifestyle).

5. Take H-Bath (Half Body Bath) once a week

The H-bath (Half Body Bath) was popularized in Korea and I was recommended to it by my oriental medicine/acupuncture doctor about a year ago . The h-bath was founded by Dr.Yoshiharu Shindo, who is a physician in Japan, and spread into Korea and China through the years. Epsom salts are made up of the compound magnesium sulfate, and they got their name because one of the earliest discoveries of magnesium and sulfate was in Epsom, England. The earliest use of salts and minerals for bathing was published in China around 2700 years BCE. Hippocrates also encouraged his fellow healers to make use of salt water to heal various ailments by immersing their patients in sea water. The ancient Greeks continued this, and in 1753 English author and physician Dr. Charles Russel published "The Uses of Sea Water" for humans for bathing for its healing capabilities.

I find the baths to be detoxifying, as you are immersed in the hottest temp you can handle (no more than 15 minutes) up to your belly button. You will find that you start to sweat profusely and all the sweat that you are sweating is toxins escaping your body. If done on a regular basis, this bath will have you feeling better, lose weight, and have more energy.

The Five R Alkaline Matrix Implementation System applied here....

Recognize: Be aware of your posture, the way you breath, how much you exercise. Keep a log of your current behaviors and make sure to note what changes you need to make.

Remove: Get rid of the bad postures, bad breathing habits, and exercise patterns.

Replenish/Reprogram: Correct the posture with the proper posture, see my guide, breath consciously fully inhaling and exhaling throughout the day, and perform regular recommended exercises that are not acid forming.

Repeat/Reconnect: Repeat the new exercise, breathing, and postural patterns regularly for 21 days.

Restore/Restart: Progress exercises as you become stronger, you will need more intensity for challenge. If you lose track, start back on the program.

Section 10:
Introduction

I find it entertaining when circling around the Pilates enthusiasts and the Yogis, since I have a background and interest in both, I am struck by how we identify ourselves. I think it is our natural inclination to belong to a group or identify with an ideal of sorts to really take a stance in the world.

In my insatiable desire to know more, I stumbled across the QiGong Method. I've tried Tai Chi but never felt the attraction toward these methods as they weren't as appealing as yoga and pilates. Simply put, it was not as vogue and sexy as the practice of Yoga and Pilates.

As some of you may be aware, my medical condition and my unrelenting desire to find answers to my condition lead me back to my roots, Sa Sang Medicine, the eastern medicine practice deep rooted in China. I've infused the macrobiotics practice from Japan and the Sa Sang theories to the Alkaline Program, especially in the Alkaline Dieting Program.

The truth is that as my body was fast deteriorating from my medical condition, I needed a way to feel normal again and regain my physical health. As an avid exercise enthusiast, the joint impacting exercises I used to love no longer was an option for me as I felt the inflammation evidenced by the pain I had post exercise. I felt defeated, however, I knew that there had to be a way to regain my physical fitness.

Yoga and Pilates were the answer to my inquiry. However, once I began to practice and learn about the Qi Gong method, I was convinced that it too was the missing piece to my journey. I believe the "exercise" often is associated with "hard work". To our mind, I think it's more enticing and pleasant to call it "movement". Our joints, muscles, and our visceral organs are in constant motion. Even at the cellular level, our movements generate energy flow, via various channels such as the lymphatic system, circulatory system, cardiovascular system, digestive, system, neurological system, and the endocrine system. In the eastern philosophy, this phenomena of Qi is defined as the life force or energy. The concept of the Qi and its meridian channels will be explained more in detail later in the Qi Gong section.

In order to understand how the YoQiLates originated, it's important to review the foundations of the three disciplines of Yoga, Qi Gong, and Pilates respectively. One thing that the three have in common is the use of the breath, postural awareness, movement, and mental focus (meditation). Some of the poses or the movements are named after various animals rooting us back to natural order and I find that the three disciplines also utilize visual imagery to an extent. Harnessing energy from both internal and the external environment is key in keeping the movements to flow and finding true self.

I will go over each discipline in brief detail and then review the practice of YoQiLates.

Section 11:
Motor Learning Theory

Since we are discussing the topic of alkaline abs as a movement, I must include this section on motor learning theory. It is my hope to establish a good foundation for you to understand your body and its capabilities.

Motor learning is a branch of science of understanding the acquisition and modification of movement. Motor learning is applicable in situations from rehabilitation to elite performance. Motor learning occurs via various feedback mechanisms--visual, tactile, auditory, and kinetic. These feedback mechanisms are necessary for the individual to be aware of their performance. Feedback can be intrinsic, coming from within the person or it can be altered, supplemented, or added feedback derived from the external sources.

Motor learning is dependent on the person's attention level. The "cognitive" stage of learning is where the attention is great because it requires one to focus. As the person begins to integrate the learning in their own bodies, the attention can then decrease. The ideal outcome of learning is to become "autonomous", which requires little to no conscious attention to perform the newly learned movement.

There are three processes that are required in the acquisition of new movement, perception, cognition, and action.

As a rehabilitation professional my primary goal is to

- Identify the faulty motor strategy that aggravates the symptoms or pain.

- Break down the motor strategy to correct the faulty pattern that is exacerbating the symptoms.

- Facilitate the correct movement pattern that does not negatively affect the symptoms.

- Practice the new strategy until the motor learning becomes efficient and autonomic.

The three primary causes of faulty movement are:

- Birth defects and anomalies can often be the cause of a variety of faulty motor learning.

- Habitual adaptations can lead to imbalances that are responsible for various faulty motor learning.

- Compensation due to injury of pain is another contributor to the faulty motor learning.

The above three potential causes of faulty motor programs need to be addressed prior to beginning any exercise programs to prevent further exacerbation and damage to the structures. For example, I often have patients with hip pain and various professionals constantly address the hip when the real problem is in the lumbar segment L4-5. It is important to treat the cause of the lesion rather than focusing on the site of the pain.

Bioenergetics

The body is comprised of the skeletal system, vascular system, muscular system, digestive system, lymphatic system, neurological system, etc. The most important system that is overlooked in the western medicine is the energetic system. Eastern medical approaches including acupuncture, herbs, acupressure, shiatsu etc are based on the energy flows as the governing force that gives vital life force to all the other systems. Similarly, yoga, pilates, and the ayurvedic medicine are also energy based. These ancient systems, which have empirically proven its effects view the body as the microcosm of the universe. For example, knee pain may be treated by addressing the energetic system of the kidneys. The weakness in the kidneys are known to make the knee joints more vulnerable and less responsive to treatment. It is important to note that it is what is unseen provides the ultimate truth and the healing power rather than what is seen that is partial and fleeting. The western philosophies are focused on the evidence based science that needs to be tangible, seen, and proven. However, the eastern philosophies provide the timeless wisdom and understanding that far exceeds our human understanding.

I've combined the understanding from the two dualities of thought and made it possible to apply the principles for our maximum benefit.

Section 12:
Yoga

Yoga originated in India. Indian's culture is among the oldest in the world. No one knows for sure how old yoga is, however, some scholars suspect that it's been around since the seventh millennium B.C. E. Yoga was first introduced to the American culture since 1893 by the Hindu monk, Swami Vivekananda.

Although modern science is validating many of the health benefits of yoga, its emergence was not very scientific at all as there was no way to objectively measure the outcome. The ancient yogis primarily used the observational power of their body to learn, explore and understand the world around them. They used various techniques to channel the breath and observed the effects.

Ancient yogis practiced sitting in the caves of the Himalayas and the ashrams in the countryside, guided by their predecessors, they were chanting and meditating. Here they learned to stretch their muscles, open the channels of their joints, manipulate their bodies in various contorted ways. They mimicked various animals and as a result, many of the postures carry the names of the animals.

This practice allowed the yogis to bring awareness to the bodies as their physiology was challenged to its limits. Breathing being the hallmark of the yoga practice, they noticed that certain poses and practices brought about increased energy. Through their practice, they were able to alter their blood pressure, body temperature, and respiration that was beyond logical understanding. This phenomena was fascinating to them. In conclusion, they learned that the movements in the practice can impact the nervous system.

Today, yoga is the mainstream of the fitness industry and appeals to a wide range of generations. Due to the various forms of yoga, it is understood that it's not for the flexible and the young, rather, that it can get you where you want to be physically. It cultivates understanding, awareness, focus, and appreciation, all things that are much more than the physical benefit. It has become popularized due to the craze by the young and the beautiful in Hollywood. It is estimated that approximately 15 million people in the United States along practice some form of yoga. I know that in the east, such as China, Korea, Japan, Taiwan, yoga is the mainstream as the celebrities have popularized this method of fitness.

To me, it's become much more than just a workout. Its where I can truly become grounded and centered. It's "me" time and with my aches and pains, I'd rather go to the yoga class over a massage any day. It liberates, detoxifies, and energized me for over a decade. My practice has evolved and it's become the time for my active meditation.

There are various forms of Yoga I want you to be aware of:

• Ashtanga (or Astanga) Yoga was founded by Sri K. Pattabhi Jois. This style of yoga is physically demanding as it involves synchronizing breathing with progressive and continuous series of postures. In the process, it produces increased heat in the body causing sweat glands to open and detoxify the muscles and the internal organs. The ultimate health benefit is improved circulation, flexibility, stamina, a long and lean body, and a calm mind. Ashtanga is an athletic yoga practice and is typically not for beginners.

• Bikram Yoga is the method of yoga that is practiced in a heated room founded by Bikram Choudhury. The practice is strenuous building muscular strength, endurance, cardiovascular health, and weight loss. This is the only yoga style that specializes in using the heated environment. I've personally enjoyed this practice for over 3 years and many beginners do come and practice, however, as a physical therapist, I feel that if not done with proper awareness and guidance, it's breeding grounds for injury. The high heat environment allows for more flexibility than in a normal room temperature, and unless the student knows to refrain from pushing too hard, one can cause micro injuries which can be devastating long term.

• Hatha Yoga is an easy-to-learn basic form of yoga that has become very popular in the United States. Hatha Yoga is the beginning of all Yoga styles. It incorporates Asanas (postures), Pranayama (breathing), meditation (Dharana & Dhyana) and kundalini (Laya Yoga) into a practice that can be used to achieve the desired outcome. The ideal way to practice the Hatha Yoga poses (asanas) is to approach the practice with proper intention, focus, and meditation. Do not overdo the asanas or try to compete with others. Your practice today is different from other days and with everyone else, make this your own connective time with yourself and learn, observe, and embrace where you are.

- Iyengar Yoga, developed by yoga master B.K.S. Iyengar more than 60 years ago. This yoga is known to promote strength, flexibility, endurance, and balance through coordinated breathing. The poses that do require precise body alignment and the poses are generally held longer than in other styles of yoga. In Iyengar, you slowly move into a pose, hold it for a minute or so, and then rest for a few breaths before stretching into another. Iyengar yoga is readily accessible to everyone because of its use of props such as yoga blocks, bolsters, straps, to aid in those who need support due to lack of strength or flexibility. Because of its slow pace, attention to detail, and use of props, Iyengar yoga is helpful especially good if you're recovering from an injury. Iyengar is one of the most popular types of yoga taught today.

- Kripalu is considered the yoga of consciousness. This gentle, introspective practice urges practitioners to hold poses to explore and release emotional and spiritual blockages. There are three stages in Kripalu yoga, stage one focuses on learning the postures and exploring your bodies abilities, stage two involves holding the postures for an extended time, developing concentration and inner awareness, and lastly, stage three is like a meditation in motion in which the movement from one posture to another arises unconsciously and spontaneously.

- Kundalini practice concentrates on awakening the energy at the base of the spine and drawing it upward. In addition to postures, a typical class will also include chanting, meditation, and breathing exercises.

- Power Yoga is the American interpretation of ashtanga yoga, a discipline that combines stretching, strength training, and meditative breathing. But power yoga takes ashtanga one step further. Many of the poses (also called postures or their Sanskrit name, asanas) resemble basic calisthenics -- push-ups and handstands, toe touches and side bends -- but the key to power yoga's sweat-producing, muscle-building power is the pace. Instead of pausing between poses as you would in traditional yoga, each move flows into the next, making it an intense aerobic workout.

- Restorative Yoga: Depending on the instructor, as the name implies, it is an easier form of yoga where healing and comfort is a priority. Typically, in a restorative yoga class you'll spend long periods of time lying on blocks, blankets and yoga bolsters - passively allowing muscles to relax.

- Sivananda Yoga: This traditional type of yoga combines postures, breathing, dietary restrictions, chanting, scriptural study, and meditation.

- Viniyoga: This type of yoga is commonly used as a therapeutic practice for people who have suffered injuries or are recovering from surgery. The practice tend to be gentle and promotes healing that is tailored to each person's body type.

- Vinyasa: Focuses on coordination of breath and movement and it is a physically active form of yoga. This type of yoga also is popularized here in the United States for its aerobic benefit.

Section 13:
Qi Gong

Qi gong is a study of energy. It is a study of the whole universe, including physics, chemistry, psychology, astrology, electricity, and medicine. It's been practiced in China for over 5000 years and is used for healing, prevention, energy channeling, and meditation.

As part of the Chinese medicine, Qi gong remains a mystery to many as it combines the mental concentration, breathing, movement, and sound to cultivate our "energy" force as it flows through the channels of the meridians of the body.

Qi means energy, air or breath, vitality, or the Universal force of life that forms all things in the universe. Gong means to use, practice, transform, activate, cultivate, or refine the energy for optimal health which balances the mind, body, spirit.

How does Qi Gong work?

Qi gong allows one to use the mind, body, and spirit to channel the life energy and allow it to flow through the body. Qi flows in two spectrums of energy called yin and yang.

Yin energy is characterized by its female, passive, spiritual tendencies such as woman, water earth, and spiritual life. Yang energy is characterized by its male, active, and physical tendencies such as man, fire, sky, and the physical body. The key is the balance and harmony between the two energies, the imbalances in the body or the universe can create a blockage in flow of energy which can ultimately lead to Dis-Ease.

It is important to understand that our body has a natural inclination to heal by way of creating balance in its natural state. It is when we impose threat to our bodies in the form of stress, unhealthy habits (diet, smoking, sedentary life), that our perfect balance gets disrupted. Our innate thermostat is set at a perfect "ease" point where everything is in perfect balance and harmony. It is when the body is imposed with external factors that our body begins to fall out of balance into the state of "Dis-ease". In the Eastern Medicine Philosophy, there is no disease, only our bodies imbalances are addressed. It's theory and application is logical, elemental, and basic utilizing the laws of the universe. The Western

Medicine is so complicated with all its scientific algorithms, research, and ICD 9 diagnosis. My dear friend and mentor, Dr. Chung (Chinese Medicine Physician) said, " in Eastern Medicine, one only needs to look at the patient to know where the imbalance lies", "in Western Medicine, with all its diagnostic tools and fancy technology, you end up with questionable diagnosis and medications that may calm the symptoms but ultimately cause the body to be at a further imbalance."

Qi gong attempts to heal the body energetically addressing the physical, mental, and the spiritual components. Trusting our natural abilities to heal ourselves, detecting the energetic blocks, and learning to remove them is the hallmark of this method.

Benefits of Qi Gong Practice

- Decreased pain

- Peace and joy

- Decreased stress and tension

- Improved metabolism, digestion, and immune function

- Balanced Yin-Yang energy

- Anti-Aging

- Mental clarity

- Improved muscle strength and flexibility

- Improved internal organ function

- Weight loss

- Decreased low back pain

- Improved circulation

- Improved neurological symptoms

- Improved Lupus and autoimmune

Is Qi Gong a religion?

Contrary to popular belief, Qi Gong is not a religion. It is really a branch of science, many Qi Gong masters in China call it "body science". You can experience the full benefit of Qi Gong even if you are Muslim, Hindu, Christian, Jewish, Taoist, or Buddhist. You will find that the practice is far from religion.

Threats that block the Qi

I. Nutrition:

- Quantity: Everything we eat should transform into energy that we can use. Anytime we consume more that our body can digest, we put the body at risk.

- Seasonal: It is a universal law that we have four seasons, we have seasonal vegetation for this reason, summer fruits and vegetables tend to be highly yang and expansive and the winter fruits and vegetables tend to be highly yin and contractive. We need to eat what is in season to supply the proper balance of energy, food is energy that we consume.

- Drink plenty of water. Often, we drink when we are thirsty, when we are thirsty, it means that we are already dehydrated. Drink room temperature water upon waking up in the morning for ultimate hydration at the start of the day.

- Prevent eating highly refined foods that are processed and infused with preservatives and additives that our bodies are not equipped to digest.

- Avoid sugar foods like donuts, chocolate bars, sodas, fruit juices sweetened with high fructose corn syrup, a popular sweetener that is highly artificial. These are just empty nutrition.

- Think of food as nourishment that heals and energizes your body. If you are eating due to emotional reasons, that means that you have a mental imbalance, read Alkaline Mind program.

- For a full content on the proper nutrition, read the Alkaline Dieting.

II. Seasonal Changes

- The earth revolves around the sun, rotating and the sun allows earth days and nights as well as seasonal changes. When the weather or the seasons change, the energetic levels and frequency of our bodies changes as well, if the body is not in harmony with the frequency of energy of the respective seasons. In eastern medicine, the seasonal changes bring energetic imbalances that directly affect our organs;

- In spring, liver problems are on the rise.

- In summer, heart problems are on the rise

- In the fall, lung problems are on the rise

- in the winter, kidney problems are on the rise.

Regular practice of QiGong allows our bodies to adjust to the changes in the energetic level. When your body in alignment and in harmony with the environmental energetic frequency, you will not have any health issues.

You are probably familiar with arthritic conditions worsening with the rainy or colder climate, due to the atmospheric pressure changes. Also with frequent rainy season as seen in Seattle makes people more prone to depression. These are the natural order, climatic changes that alter the energy levels that ultimately affect the health of the living beings.

III. Environment

The environment plays a critical role to our health. As the industrial revolution is at its peak causing more pollutants in the air and the water, we are noticing increased incidences of allergic reactions and autoimmune conditions.

The energy from the earth, sun, and the moon has an impact on the creatures that occupy the planet earth, including humans. I'm sure you've heard of Feng Shui, it is becoming more popular all over the world due to its positive effect. The underlying premise of Feng Shui functions under the assumption that every object possesses its own energetic field. You can learn that the energy level of the house can be altered simply by positioning the furniture in such a way to enhance the flow of the energy.

IV. Pharmacology

Western medicine relies heavily on the pharmaceuticals. Infact, it is very common practice to go to a physician and walk out with a magic pill to alleviate the symptoms when in reality, the underlying issue was not relieved.

If you read the side effect label of all prescription drugs, you'll understand the serious impact the medication has by altering the yin-yang balance.

V. Musculoskeletal Trauma

Any injuries can block the Qi, it's your body's effort to heal the site of the injury. Such traumas can create blocks to other areas of the body, impacting the wellness of your whole being.

VI. Emotional Disturbances

Emotions have a significant impact in the natural flow of Qi. In Chinese medicine, over-reaction can cause imbalance in the heart meridian, anger/anxiety can cause an imbalance in the liver, fear can cause disturbance in the kidney meridian, depression can impact the lung energy, and too much thinking can cause a blockage in the stomach and the pancreas.

Taoistic ancient wisdom advises to stay even keel to keep the yin and yang in perfect balance to promote health and healing.

There are three principles that set the foundation for an effective Qi-Gong practice.

• Meditation: Use your consciousness to go into the emptiness where thoughts ultimately cease or greatly diminish and sensory connections to our bodies fade. This allows us to be in a state of pure energy where we are one with the universal energy. Our bodies are naturally inclined to be in this emptiness, for example, when we sleep we are relaxed and peaceful. We are able to bring our body to the state of emptiness where we can take rest, allowing our blocked Qi to flow and recirculate in our bodies. The deeper you go into this state of emptiness, the better your healing abilities will become. The longer you stay in the emptiness, the faster your channels will open and stay open and the more power you will have to use your Qi.

• Simplicity: Qi Gong can be very intimidating and complicated. However Qi Gong in its fundamental form is very basic and simple. It is not necessary to learn complicated movements to open channels and release blockages, the most powerful techniques are usually the simplest.

• Use Consciousness: Consciousness is not the same as your conscious mind. Your consciousness is the infinite part of you that is able to connect with the higher power, the universal power. It is the direct connections to the emptiness, the source of all creation, where we can connect with the infinite wisdom, power, and energy. Our consciousness is always at work, sending us energy and messages, but we must quiet our mind and relax our bodies to receive them. When practicing Qi Gong, we use sensation of the body to feel the flow of Qi and our conscious mind to influence the flow. Positive thoughts, for example, encourage health and rapidly direct Qi in optimal ways. Negative thoughts on the other hand, block the energy channels and create sickness. As you practice, you will come to realize that the mental power is more powerful than the physical power.

There are three elements of the Qi Gong exercises:

I. Breathing: Deep, slow, and controlled breathing is the most important element. There is grown medical evidence that people with fewer breaths per minute are overall healthier than those who breath more rapidly. The most important systems in the body is the nervous system. The nervous system controls the information being transmitted through the body via the nerves, arteries, hormones, enzymes, neurotransmitters, etc. Blockages in the nervous system can negatively affect the essential communication that is necessary for health and wellness. In Qi Gong you will practice "energy breathing", a two step process that allows the yin and yang energy of the body join together.

Step 1: Breathing through the skin

As you inhale through your nose, concentrate your mind   on breathing through your skin and the universal energy coming through to give life to every cell in your body.   As you exhale, also through your nose, visualize any sickness leaving your body leaving you with a sense of vitality and healing.

Step 2: Access Qi

As you inhale, draw in your navel, and as you exhale, loosen your lower stomach and let it out a little. Allow this to occur naturally, simply relax and let the breath "flow" effortlessly. Note that the upper part of the body belongs to yang energy and the lower part of the body belongs to yin energy. Typically the energy coming in through inhaling is yin and the energy expelled through exhaling is yang. The two energies then communicate with each other and balance in the body.

2. Postures

Posture and movements are important because they help to open the energy channels in the body. It is simple to open the energy channel, for example, opening of the hands help to open the six energy channels that begin in the hands. This includes the lung and the large intestine channels, which begin in the thumb, and the heart channels which begin in the middle and the pinky fingers.

Postures in and of themselves can give immediate benefit. When you have a headache, cough, or stuffy nose, you can relieve the symptoms simply by holding your hands above your head for 5 minutes. Also when you have a bloody nose on the left, by raising the right hand above the head for a minute, you can help to stop the bloody nose. These simple techniques are effective because raising your hands open the lunch channels, heart channels, and stomach channels, many of which run through the nose area. By replenishing the energy to these area, the symptoms disappear.

3.   Harness your Mind/Use Visualization

Our brain is very powerful, yet, it is proven that we humans only use partial capacity, typically 2-10%. If we apply an additional 1% to the health of our bodies, we will experience miracles. Growing body of evidence proves that our minds can do wonders in our physiology by the way of altering the yin-yang energy channels and directing the hormones, neurotransmitters, enzymes, etc. Our minds have the capability to achieve anything; the problem is with our ego that are like gate keepers to limit our ability. This is because of our "conditioned" mind through our childhood and experiences that shaped our minds, we are more inclined to be safe and even though our "shaped" mind does not serve us well, we are "conditioned" to keep ourselves where we feel familiar and safe. One helpful way to free our mind to reach higher limits is to meditate on the powerful phrase.

" My spirit is greater than me, the universal energy is one with my spirit and therefore, the universal energy supplies my body with perpetual energy and power."

5 Keys To Success

1.   Faith: Life is divided into two parts: the material life that includes our physical body and the spiritual life. It is important to note that most sicknesses start in our spiritual life and manifest physically into symptoms. You will find it helpful to trust your soul and the universal energy. In the western world, we have tendency to rely on the healers and the doctors to facilitate our healing and we give up our power over to them. However, it is

important to know that no one can help us to heal unless we want to be healed. Cultivate awareness and you will be on your way to develop trust and faith, which are the essential ingredients to healing.

2. Unrelenting Confidence

The most successful people of the world has unstoppable confidence. Follow the ways to express and cultivate your own self confidence.

- Embrace your sickness as your teacher and friend. An illness often relates to how you have been conducting your life. Have you been in touch with nature? Have you taken the time to cultivate awareness and healing? What about the dietary practices? When you are sick, it is your body trying to communicate to you that you are out of balance so listen, reflect, and then correct.

- Consider the sickness as a positive learning, listen to your inner voice, learn from it to understand your life, and you will be a happier and healthier person.

- Accept the responsibility that you have the power to heal yourself. We have the innate ability as a gift, the more you use them the more you will become a powerful healer.

- Have faith in your heart that one day, through continuous practice, you will get well.

Remember that the blockages and illnesses are not formed in a day. Sometimes, it takes time to release the blockages and find health again. They also stay inside your body as a teacher to teach you how to regain your own health.

3. Use your spiritual connection to the higher power.

In my case, it is my Jesus Christ, the Son of God. You can use the general "universal" power, the creator, whatever your beliefs are, call on the help of the greater source of power. In the east, it can be Lao Tzu, Buddha, whoever you hold high respect for. As you meditate, ask for their guidance, when you are able to go into that empty space, you can get connected but it is only when you are free from the distraction of your own mind.

4. Concentration

The idea of concentration when meditating is very different. Meditation focus involves you bringing energy inside your body and focusing on one point. At the same time, use your mind to feel energy moving in all parts of your body. Relax yourself into a state of being so that you get yourself in the state of nothingness.

5. Visualization

Visualization is very powerful way to enhance your mediation and self-healing. You may want to visualize you blockage in the kidney, bone, pain, or tumor transformed into air and coming out of your body. You may even want to visualize black smoke that symbolizes pain and disease leaving your body into the universe, freeing your body from all harm. Feel free to experiment with whatever works for you.

Visualization is energy, it ignites a chemical process in the body and through those means, it can meet the needs of the body and to help the body to open up and heal its blockages.

Don't give yourself a hard time in the beginning if you are having a difficult time visualizing, just trust that the energy is working because it is.

The Secret Happiness and Joy

The power of the Qi Gong is in unconditional love, forgiveness, and kindness. The benefit of Qi Gong is that through its practice, you can learn to understand your life and the freedom of life, physically and spiritually. You will find that the fear, struggle, anxiety, anger, hatred, jealousy disappears and happiness, love, kindness, and forgiveness resides in you. This will be when you know that you've achieved the connectedness with the practice and it will only improve with time.

Remember life is happiness. You can gain happiness by giving your love and forgiveness to others.

Practice YoQiLates every day to benefit from the very essence of Qi Gong. It will indeed help you cultivate awareness, love, kindness, healing, and happiness. You will find that your life will present more opportunities for success, friendships, and happiness, keep your heart open to the emerging possibilities, the possibilities that you've lived without in the past. As you continue to connect with the universal power and energy, you will find balance in yin and yang in your body and you will find greater health, joy, and happiness.

Balanced Exercise: Precision, Alignment, and Breathing

"I must be right. Never an aspirin. Never injured a day in my life. The whole country, the whole world, should be doing my exercises. They'd be happier."
- Joseph Hubertus Pilates, in 1965, age 86.

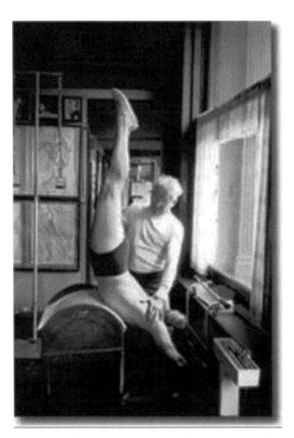

Over the past 15 years, awareness about the benefits of Pilates as an exercise has exploded. Pilates is a method of exercise and physical movement designed to elongate, strengthen, and balance the body. With systematic practice of specific exercises coupled with focused breathing patterns, Pilates has proven itself invaluable not only as a fitness endeavor, but also as an important adjunct to professional sports training and physical rehabilitation for all people.

Widely embraced by the professional dance community during much of the 20th century, the names of the unique exercises -- "elephant," "swan", the language -- "pull navel to spine, and breeaaaathe," and the look -- bright-eyed, refreshed, light on the feet, perfectly postured, buoyant-without-necessarily-sweating, are now commonly found in fitness classes, physical therapy offices, corporate retreats, luxury spas and wellness centers today. With the aging of our population and the increasing trend toward mindful, moderate health practices, Pilates is in increasing demand with a wait list for the classes at the YMCA, and in your local public schools--reshaping the fitness ideals of our next generation.

Practiced consistently, Pilates provides numerous benefits. Increased lung capacity and circulation through deep, healthy breathing is a primary focus. Strength and flexibility, particularly of the abdomen, arms, legs, and the back muscles, coordination - both neurological, muscular, and mental, are key components in an effective Pilates program. Posture, balance, and core strength are all addressed and inevitably improved. Bone density and joint health improve, and many experience positive body awareness and posture for the first time. Pilates teaches balance and control of the body, and that learned skill spills over into other areas of one's life.

Joseph Pilates, demonstrating the importance of his unique exercise equipment.

Around 1914, Joseph Pilates was a performer and a boxer living in England, with the outbreak of WWI, was placed under forced internship along with other German nationals in Lancaster, England. There he taught fellow camp members the concepts and exercises developed over 20 years of self-study and apprenticeship in yoga, Zen, and ancient Greek and Roman physical regimens. It was at this time that he began devising the system of original exercises known today as "matwork", or exercises done on the floor. He called this regimen "Contrology", meaning 'the science of control'. A few years later, he was transferred to another camp on the Isle of Man, where he became a nurse/caretaker to the many internees struck with disease and physical injury from the war. Here, he began devising equipment to rehabilitate the "patients" that were under his care, taking springs from the beds and rigging them to create spring resistance and "movement" for the bedridden. In a way, Pilates equipment today is not much different than that of yesterday. Spring tension, straps to hold feet or hands, supports for back, neck and shoulder are as important now as they were then. Because of the remarkable nature of the equipment to both challenge and support the body as it learns to move more efficiently, the inimitably designed pieces truly act as a complement to the challenging "mat work" exercises.

Clara Pilates
While Joe was the outspoken force behind his method, his wife Clara quietly incorporated his concepts and exercises in ways that benefited more seriously ill or injured clients. Her approachable style and special techniques spawned a dedicated lineage of teachers whose work flows through and uniquely colors the landscape of the Pilates method today. It is perhaps because of Clara that Pilates is clearly recognized as a positive form of movement-based exercise that truly can be tailored to any level of not just fitness, but also of health.

Joseph Pilates, on natural movement and the period of time taken to study the human body.

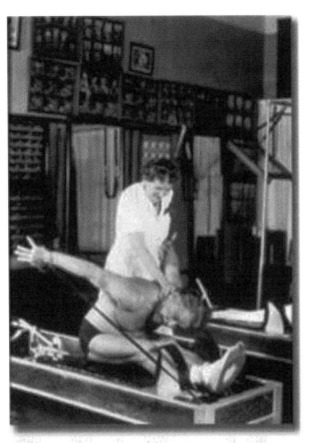

"Everything should be smooth, like a cat. The exercises are done lying, sitting, kneeling, etc, to avoid excessive strain on the heart and lungs."

First generation Pilates teachers, who knew Joe, maintain that Clara and Joseph would be very happy and proud of the popularity and growth of Pilates. However, it is less clear how he might feel about the influx of "quickie trainings" available for would-be instructors wanting to be trained in a weekend or two. Joe worked at length with his own teachers, allowing them to assist and then finally teach after sometimes as long as 2 or 3 years of training and apprenticeship. He was quoted as saying, "Remember Rome was not built in a day.", and "Patience and persistence are vital qualities in the ultimate successful accomplishment of any worthwhile endeavor." He was truly beyond his time.

While excellent training programs exist in the marketplace today, some are clearly condensed and homogenized, producing less-than-optimally qualified teachers. Prices for classes range from $10-$20 for group mat sessions, to upwards of $50-$100 for one hour of one-on-one instruction utilizing the full repertoire of Pilates equipment. Comprehensively, competently trained and knowledgeable teachers are the essential element in realizing one's potential as a client, and enjoying the process of learning Pilates. By the early 1960's Joe and Clara were training many of the New York dancers. George Balanchine invited Joseph to train his young ballerinas at the New York City Ballet. Several of his first generation teachers began to open their own studios after his death and his work began to propagate. Today, there are numerous Pilates training programs worldwide and approximately 5 million Americans practice Pilates and the numbers continue to grow.

Section 15:
YoQiLates

YoQiLates is a complete movement method to energize, heal, and tone your body. Unlike the no pain no gain model of the fitness industry, I've created this revolutionary method with improving your overall health. The organic acids, lactic acids, that are produced via hard core exercise program create an acid environment in your body causing unnecessary stress with onset of various symptoms such as:

- Lack of energy, fatigue, loss of physical tone and lack of motivation, heaviness in the limbs, and hopelessness.
- Cold hands and feet.
- Tendency to get infections.
- Loss of drive, joy and enthusiasm.
- Depression.
- Nervousness, agitation without cause, hyperactivity, sensitivity to high-pitched noises and easily stressed.
- Pale complexion.
- Headaches.
- Teary eyes.
- Conjunctivitis.
- Swelling of the and eyelids.
- Acidic saliva.
- Loose teeth.
- Inflamed, sensitive gums.
- Mouth ulcers.
- Cracks at the corners of the lips.
- Recurring infections of throat and tonsils.
- Sensitivity to hot, cold or acidic foods.
- Pain in the nerves of the teeth.
- Excess or lack of stomach acid.
- Acid reflex.
- Gastritis.
- Ulcers.
- Nails are thin and split and break easily.
- Hair looks dull, has split ends, and falls out.
- Dry skin.

- Skin tends to be irritated in regions where there are heavy concentrations of sweat.
- Hives.
- Leg cramps and spasms.

If you or anyone you know are suffering from number of above symptoms, you may want to consider the practice of YoQiLates.

YoQiLates combines the three practices; Yoga, QiGong, and Pilates. The method sequence integrates the three practices seamlessly to optimize the benefit of each practices.
Since in the previous sections I reviewed the theory and foundation of each practice, I will only discuss the combined method of the YoQiLates.

Before I go any further, it is important to go over the meridians in the human body. The meridians are considered to be primary "Qi" channels. Your body has twelve channels, which in Chinese medicine, it is considered to be like rivers of "Qi".
The ends of each channel is associated with one of the twelve organs in the body, while the other end is connected to the toe or fingers (six channels are connected to the fingers and the other six are connected to the toes).
There are Qi vessels in the body which can be compared to batteries and capacitors in an electrical system. Batteries store and then release electrical current, and capacitors regulate the electrical current in the same way that the vessels regulate the Qi in your channels and organs.
In order for us to be optimally healthy, the Qi must flow smoothly and continuously in the channels. However, we often have blockages as the blockages can be caused by poor eating habits, injuries, and the inevitable degeneration that occurs with old age.
YoQiLates is much more than a physical practice. It is a spiritual, physical, and mental practice that will allow you to get in touch with your true potential for health and healing.

There are seven core principles of YoQiLates:
I. Intention: It is important that the one practicing YoQiLates is aware that at the core, every system in our bodies at the cellular level is programmed for optimal health. It is when we are out of sync with our universal life force or "Qi" we are subject to disease. Set your intention to heal and be clear about what you want to accomplish with the practice of YoQiLates. Setting intentions prior to embarking on a journey or practice will dictate the outcome of your efforts. Let it be aligned

with your core desire to heal and be at peace each time you practice. Remind yourself of what you want to get out of each practice.

II. Yin-Yang Balance: Our aim in the practice of YoQiLates is to ensure that we have perfect balance in our body. Yin and Yang are the natural dualities that exist in this universe, such as (man-woman, hot-cold, north-south, dark-light, low-high, water-fire, life-death, etc.). Yin and yang cannot exist without the other and either one is good or bad, it just is. This duality exists in everything from foods, weather, relationships, and it even exists inside ourselves. In the Chinese culture, yin and yang are known to transform each other: like an undertow in the ocean, every advance is complemented by a retreat, and every rise transforms into a fall. Thus, a seed will sprout from the earth and grow upwards towards the sky—an intrinsically yang movement. Then, when it reaches its full potential height, it will fall, yin movement. It is our aim to practice balance of yin and yang in all areas of our practice and as you progress, it will overflow into other areas of your life.

III. Agility: Movement is absolutely necessary for Qi to flow. In the west, it is common to consider movement as "exercise", the no pain no gain mentality where the balance in our systems are challenged to a point of damaging our health and our physiological structure. In YoQiLates, we will practice moving with agility. We are designed to move and move with ease. Due to the nature of our technological culture and sedentary life, moving is laborious. We've become too yin, too contracted, tight, stiff, and difficult to move. If practiced regularly, you will find that movement will be a breeze again. Practice of YoQiLates regularly can reverse arthritis, slow aging process, improve flexibility, agility, strength, and mental focus.

IV. Qi Energy: The nature of Qi in the human body, we need to understand where to Qi originates. Something cannot come from nothing, so Qi (energy) must come from matter. It is important to note that the matter is a physical form of energy and the energy is an "unlocked potential" of matter. For example, when we eat food, through the biochemical reaction, we transform the food into the Qi. We are dealing with two forms of energy, the electromagnetic energy and the potential energy. Qi typically moves from the area of higher potential to the area of lower potential and this is occurring naturally and automatically to bring your system into balance. This Qi will be harnessed, strengthened, and most importantly circulated to ensure that there are no blockages in the meridians of our bodies.

V. Focus: The series of postures will align your physical body and the mental focus to also overflow into other areas of your life. The method of YoQiLates requires you to have complete mental focus and intention during the practice to enable you to harness your healing abilities and allow your body to succumb to its natural tendencies again. This focus will allow your body to reconnect with its intrinsic thermostat and reset its internal setting to optimize the healing, health, and vitality.

VI. Breathing: There are two sources of "essence" to supply your body's needs. They are air and food. As these two are absorbed into our bodies, they are converted into Qi. Breathing is an important part of the YoQiLates practice and also for general health, which is well documented in research. It is important to understand the respiration cycle of inhalation and exhalation. In order for the air to reach the lungs and be pushed out, the muscles around the lungs and the diaphragm must expand and contract. During this process, the fresh oxygen will mix with the blood in the lungs and the blood will release carbon dioxide via exhalation. The diaphragm is moving up and down during the cycle of respiration and it massages the internal organs and increase the Qi circulation throughout the organ systems and the body. It is important to note that the brain needs far more oxygen than the rest of our body, this is why when you lack oxygen, you can feel dizzy, heavy, and are unable to think clearly. In the west, the breathing becomes shallower and shallower as one gets older, especially with the preoccupation with technology, working on the computer and gadgets, decreasing our movement during the day. In YoQiLates, you will learn to regulate and control your breathing pattern by consciously breathing with intent. You will notice improved energy, vitality, memory, and health.

VII. Posture: As a physical therapist, I regard posture highly in any treatment protocol. If you are not properly postured, you will have blockages in Qi, compensation of muscles, arthritis, and imbalances. Think of your body as a car and the tires, suspension, and the alignment of the tires as your limbs. What would happen over time if your tires are not rotated regularly, alignment not checked, and the suspension broken? That's right; its good smooth ride will be compromised before long. In YoQiLates, posture and alignment will be emphasized to have your organ systems work more efficiently, improving your breathing ability, optimizing Qi (energy) flow, and helping you to be lean and toned.

Key Postures:

There are the fundamental key postures for the practice of YoQilates. It is important to keep in mind that the practice of YoQilates is intended to open up the meridian channels in the body and cultivate your spiritual energy for optimal healing and health. Following are the basic set of poses for the purpose of the book. The complete practice involves both dynamic flow (yang energy), and static (yin energy). Remember that structurally we are all different; therefore, don't be discouraged if you are not able to get into the poses easily in the beginning.

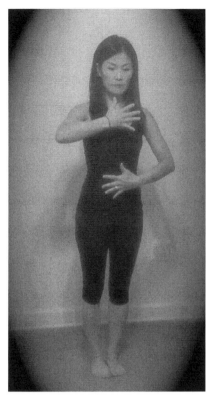

• Yin-Yang Balance: The upper part of the torso above the navel is considered to be "yang" and the lower part of the body below the navel is considered to be "yin". This poses attempts to balance the energy of both yin and yang. Right hand is more of the "yang energy" held near the heart and the left hand is more of the "yin energy" held below the navel. Breath consciously, imagine a transparent energy column in the middle of your torso emanating light through the whole spinal column. Take a deep inhale in and exhale, continue to take long deep breaths for a cycle of 10. Visualize the universal energy flowing into your body with every inhalation healing your cells and the toxic negative energy leaving your body with every exhalation.

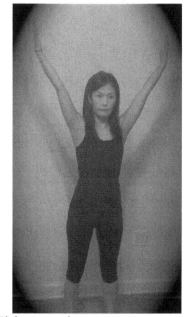

• Mountain Pose: Keep the fingers open at times as this enables the meridian channels to remain open. With inhalation, bring your arms up and over head and with exhalation, bring your arms down to the mountain pose. This pose is very energizing, repeat for a cycle of 5 and you will feel the energy vibrating throughout your body.

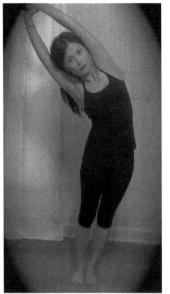

• Sidebend: First take a hold of your left wrist with your right hand and pull straight up keeping the shoulders down and bend over to the right side keeping the sides of the waist long and elongated. Take a breath in and feel the rib cage expand even further and exhale, do not let the chest collapse. Breath 5 cycles on this side and repeat the same on the opposite side. This pose allows the lungs on both sides to really take in the fresh oxygen allowing the chest cavity to expand fully. The Qi is then energized and circulated and blocked Qi will be open.

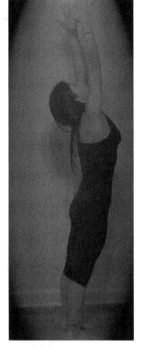

• Back Bend: Stretch up in a mountain pose and raise your arms overhead with slight back bend. Allow your exhale to lower and ground your feet, imaging that you have deep roots that are keeping you down firmly. Allow your inhale to lift up from your spine and imagine your spine getting longer and you getting taller.

This spine stimulates and opens all energy channels and helps to stimulate the nervous system, improve posture by realigning your spine, promotes kidney function, and the digestive system.

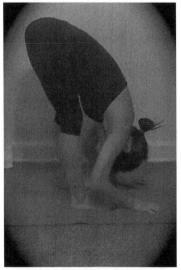

Forward Bend: Begin in mountain pose and as you exhale, bend forward and allow your shoulders to relax and ease into the bend. Take deep breath in and exhale into the bend further. Repeat 5 breath cycles. This is a pose where the head is below your heart and allows the blood to rush into your head, opening the meridian channels and rejuvenating the yang part of the body with oxygenated blood. Keep your knees slightly bent if you have tight hamstrings or low back pain. It's a good idea to keep deeply rooted through your feet and bear weight evenly between the legs.

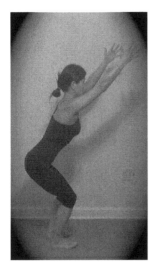

• Chair: When starting out, keep the feet shoulder width apart, as you get stronger and more centered, keep the feet together. From mountain pose inhale your arms up and overhead and ease down as if you are sitting in a chair. It is important to keep your knees behind your toes as you can compromise the knee joint otherwise. Take deep inhale in and exhale out for 5 breath cycles. It helps to keep focused on one object in the room. As you get stronger, you can be at 90 degrees at the knee joint by sitting further down, in the beginning it's not important how far you go down. It is important to keep shoulders down and spine aligned. You will feel the burn in your thighs. This pose stimulates the heart, diaphragm, and the abdominal organs.

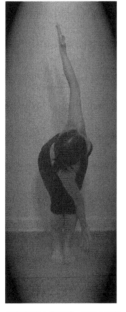

• Twisted Chair: In the beginning, start with your feet shoulder width apart and go into the chair pose. Rotate your spine by bringing the right arm down to the left side of your left foot and keep the left arm up toward the ceiling. Keep your chest lifted and take a deep breath in and out for 5 cycles. It is important to keep your pelvis square toward the front to keep your spine centered and aligned. This pose opens the energy channels in the spine, improves digestion, and alleviate aches and pain in the low back and the hips.

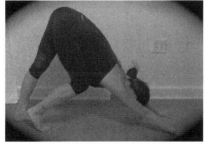

• Down Dog wagging tail: The hands should remain open to allow the energy to flow, "plug" your entire hand fully into the ground at all times, the feet are hips width apart and bend right knee on inhale and exhale and repeat with the left knee bent. Visualize your tail wagging side to side to open up your spine and allow energy flow. Keep your neck completely relaxed, as with all the other exercises, repeat for 5 complete breaths on each side.

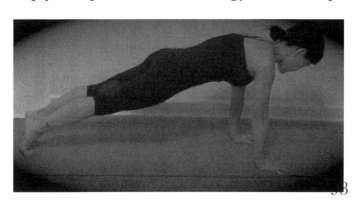

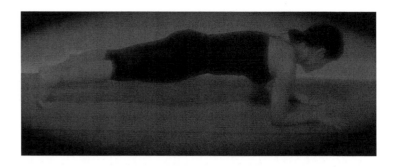

• Plank: Keeping your shoulder 90 degrees from your torso, keep your torso straight, neck relaxed. Two versions are shown here, with the arms straight and on your forearms. Try both, you'll find that the pose on your forearms are a bit more challenging. Breath in and out for five complete slow cycles. This posture keeps the core stable, elongates the body and lengthens the neck.

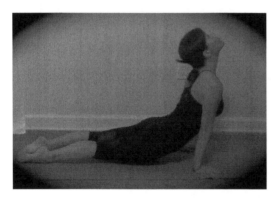

• Upward Dog : Start by lying face down, legs should be long with a feeling of extension through the length of the toes and spread hips-widths apart. Bend your elbows and place palms flat on the floor, fingers spread wide. Keep the hands "plugged" into the floor for stability. Press firmly down through the top of the feet; top of all 10 toes should be on the floor. Pull up looking up toward the ceiling or straight ahead. The only contact with the floor should be tops of the feet and the whole hand, rest of the body lifted. Breath in and out slow full cycles of breath for 5 cycles. This pose will strengthen the spine, arms and wrists, stimulate the abdominal organs, improve posture, and improve Qi energy flow.

Seated (Yin) Poses

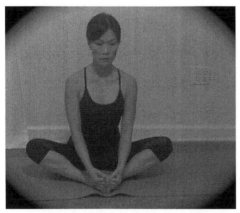

• Butterfly: Sit with your spine straight and legs spread out. Bend your knees and bring your feet toward the pelvis, the soles of the feet should touch each other. Grab your feet tightly with your hands, make an effort to bring the heels close to you as possible. Take a deep inhale and out, press the thighs and knees downward toward the floor, making an effort to press them down. Lean forward and remain in this pose for 3 minutes. This pose helps to loosen the hip energy channel which helps with intestines and bowel movements. This pose also offers relief from menstrual and menopause symptoms.

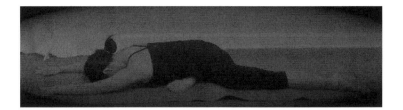

• Pigeon: Start on all fours, slide the right knee forward toward the right hand, slide the left leg back as far as possible. Keep your hips square to the floor, if your hips are not square, it can pose stress to your back. To get full release, breath once cycle and release your upper body over the knee, remain in this pose breathing in and out for 3 minutes, and repeat on the other side. This pose helps to stimulate your internal organs, stretch your hips, and can help with emotional instability. This pose also is excellent to release the blocked energy in the hips.

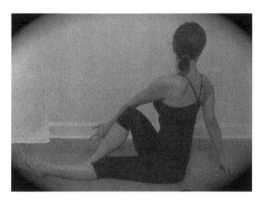

• Twist: Sit with your legs forward and bend the right knee, bring your left elbow to the outside of the right knee and life your torso up and twist, breath in and on exhale go into the twist a bit more, stay in this pose for 3 minutes and repeat on the other side. Make sure to breath consciously. This pose stimulates the kidneys, improves energy to the internal organs, and energizes the spine.

• Forward bend: If you have tight hamstrings, it is best to use a bolster between your knees. Sit straight up with your legs straight in front of you. Lift up your

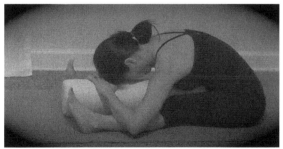

torso and forward bend over your legs if you have the flexibility, and completely relax into the pose with every cycle of breath, making sure to relax your shoulders and arms. As mentioned earlier, feel free to use a bolster, important thing is to be able to feel the stretch in the back of the legs and are able to ease and relax into the pose. Consciously breath for 3 minutes. This pose levels out the yin energy, calms the brain and relieve stress and depression. This pose is known to stimulate the Qi energy of the liver, kidneys, ovaries, and uterus. This pose also helps with digestion, soothes anxiety, and calms the headaches.

On all Fours

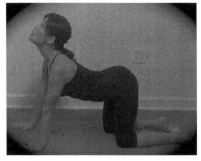

• Cat/Camel: Start with your hands and knees on the floor, hip widths apart. Bring your arms right below your shoulder, keeping the hands wide open for energy flow. Drop your spine and look up as you draw the shoulders down, tail bone is angled up toward the ceiling. Then tuck the tail under and round out the spine looking down at your navel, really engaging your abdominal muscles. Make sure to "plug" down your hands and knees to the floor to enable this motion to occur in the spine. Mindfully breathe in when you look up and exhale as you look down repeat 5 complete cycle breaths. This pose allows for energy releases in the spine. Both yin and yang balance is promoted, expands the rib cage, and relieves the stagnation and stiffness in the lower back. This pose also improves the circulation to the brain.

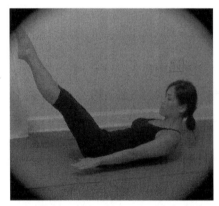

• Supine Hundred: on your back with your legs bent in table top position with your shins and ankles parallel to the floor. Inhale and then exhale as you bring your head up with your chin down and using your abdominal muscles, curl your neck and upper spine up gazing down at your flat navel. Keep the shoulders drawn down and arms long by your side. Stay here and inhale for 10 and exhale for 10 short breaths. This exercise allows for the respiration cycles to release and absorb Qi energy and strengthens the core stability and improve posture.

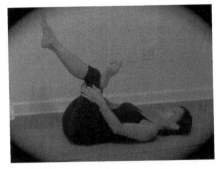

• Trunk rotation stretch: Lie on your back and bend the right knee up to your chest and bring over the left leg and twist over to the left side. Right arm extends out to the right side and look over to the right. Stay in this pose for 3 minutes mindfully breathing full cycles and relaxing into this pose. Then repeat on the opposite side and stay there for 3 minutes. This pose is excellent for releasing the vital Qi energy in the spine, stimulating all internal organs, improving respiration, and has an alkalizing effect in the respiration.

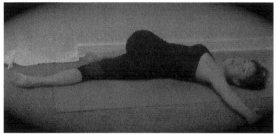

• Eye of the needle (piriformis stretch): Lie on your back and bring the right ankle just above the left knee and reach down with your arms between your legs and bring the left knee toward your chest by pulling up with your arms. Try to flatten the whole spine and feel the intense stretch into the right hip. Breath in and out mindfully and hold here for 3 minutes and repeat on the opposite side. By opening the hips, this pose allows for easing low back pain, improving circulation in your legs, improve the way you walk, decrease stress and anxiety. Hips are intimately connected to many meridians and it often is the site of "blockage". This release allows for the energy to be rebalanced between the Yin and Yang.

• Prone Cobra: Start by lying on your stomach on a level surface. The legs can be either together or hip widths apart, spread your hands on the floor just under your shoulders and hug your elbows into your rib cage. Inhale and straighten your arms and lift your chest from the floor, activating your abdominal muscles to protect your back. Stay grounded by having your hands firmly rooted into the floor and breathing long deep breaths in and out mindfully for 5 cycles. Slowly release and turn your head to the right and relax. This backbend posture improves your postur e, mood, energizes the heart, stimulates the abdominal organs and the kidneys.

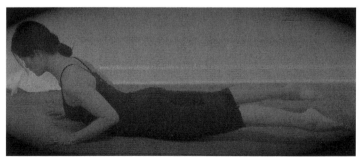

• Prone Extension: Start lying on your stomach and activate your abdominals by drawing the belly button to the spine, arms are close to your body, hands are spread out just under your shoulders. Activate the core and the legs and lift your chest up , gazing straight ahead while you also lift both legs. Don't worry about the height, if you feel uncomfortable lifting the legs off the floor, just straighten them with the pointed toes to ensure that the legs are "active". Breath in and out full cycles for 5 and release down and turn your neck to the left and relax completely and breath. This posture also allows for energy to flow through the spine, strengthens both the back, core, and the legs improving the posture.

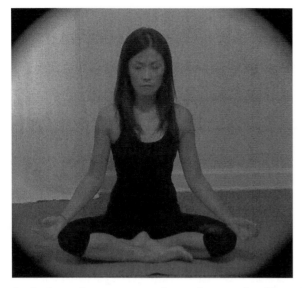

• Seated meditation: This process is the most beneficial; initially it's natural to have a difficult time quieting your mind. The more you practice this, the better you will become and you will be amazed at the benefit that you'll have in your body as well as in your life.

The meditative process opens the energy channels by developing mental concentration and controlled breathing. To begin, sit with your legs cross as in the picture or you may want to sit in a chair keeping your spine nice and tall, palms should face up. Keep the tip of the tongue on the roof of the mouth as this allows for the energy channels to remain open.

We have numerous energy channels in our bodies; we will attempt to open those channels with our mental efforts by way of imagery.

Concentrate your mind on the lower dantian (just below the navel), visualize your own energy emanating from your body as a bright light shining out from the navel. Take long and purposeful breaths in and out and continue imagining this light from your lower dantian extending through your whole body, clearing the way for the energy to flow and healing every cell and part of your body. Keep visualizing anything that may come up, taking deep breaths in and out. Tell yourself that "all my channels are open and flowing, there are no blockages, but a radiant healing light that is infusing and healing my body. Repeat this process continuing to focus on the light in your body. Start out for at least 15 minutes and can build your time up to however long. Meditation and its benefits on health and wellness have been well documented and in our culture of information overload, we are all seeking ways to quiet our minds. I recommend that you practice the whole sequence described here every day for 40 days and journal your progress. It is my belief that after 40 days, you will not want to stop as you will have transformed your body and your mind.

Complete sequence and progression of the practice of YoQiLates will be available both in print and in video on my website. Visit, bestlifeblueprint.com

Section 16:
Breathing

The importance of Breathing:

Breathing is important for two reasons. It allows supply of oxygen to our vital organs and body, which is essential for our survival. The second function of breathing is that it allows waste products and toxins to be detoxified from the body.

Oxygen is the most vital nutrient for our bodies. It is essential for the health of the brain, nerves, glands and internal organs. We can do without food for weeks and without water for days, but without oxygen, we will die within a few minutes. If the brain does not gets proper supply of this essential nutrient, it will result in the degradation of all vital organs in the body.

The brain requires more oxygen than any other organ. If it doesn't get enough, the result is mental sluggishness, negative thoughts and depression and, eventually, vision and hearing decline.

Oxygen Purifies

One of the major secrets of vitality and rejuvenation is a purified blood stream. The quickest and most effective way to purify the blood stream is by taking in extra supplies of oxygen from the air we breathe. Daily breathing exercises are the most effective methods ever devised for saturating the blood with extra oxygen.

Oxygen stirs up the waste products (toxins) from the body, as well as recharging the body's batteries (the solar plexus). In fact, most of our energy requirements come not from food but from the air we breathe.

By purifying the blood stream, every part of the body benefits, as well as the mind. Your complexion will become clearer and brighter and wrinkles will begin to fade away. Most importantly, you will be rejuvenated and your weight loss efforts will be more effective.

With the current technological culture where we are sedentary and fixated in front of the computer, we've become shallow breathers as a society. This is true especially in the developed countries throughout the world.

Reasons for shallow breathing:

a. We live in a fast paced world; our physiological patterns follow this pattern. The increasing stress of modern living makes us breathe more quickly and less deeply. Due to increased stress, our emotional response is very dramatic, we tend to get excited easily, are angered easier, and we ultimately suffer from anxiety. These negative emotional states affect the rate of breathing, causing it to be fast and shallow.

b. Modern technology and automation reduces our need for physical activity. There is less need to breathe deeply, so we develop the shallow breathing habit.

c. We are working indoors more and more. This increases our exposure to pollution. As a result, the body innately inhales less air to protect itself from pollution. The body just takes in enough air to tick over.

d. As we go through life, these bad breathing habits we picked up become part of our life. Unless we do something to reverse these habits, we can suffer permanent problems.

e. The good news is that these are reversible. The bad news is that before we can change these habits, we should recognize and accept that our behavior needs to be changed. This means that we see for ourselves the benefits of good breathing techniques.

Deep breathing exercises and stretching of muscles, especially those primarily concerned with controlling inhaling and exhaling, should be learned and practiced daily. Participation in cardiovascular exercises will be beneficial, for example, walking, jogging, and playing recreational sports.

Benefits of Breathing

1. Improvement in the quality of the blood due to its increased oxygenation in the lungs. This aids in the elimination of toxins from the system.

2. Increase in the digestion and assimilation of food.

3. Improvement in the health of the nervous system, including the brain, spinal cord, nerve centers and nerves.

4. Rejuvenation of the glands, especially the pituitary and pineal glands. The brain has a special affinity for oxygen, requiring three times more oxygen than does the rest of the body.

5. Rejuvenation of the skin. The skin becomes smoother and a reduction of facial wrinkles occurs.

6. The movements of the diaphragm during the deep breathing exercise massage the abdominal organs - the stomach, small intestine, liver and pancreas.

7. Deep, slow breathing assists in weight control. If you are overweight, the extra oxygen burns up the excess fat more efficiently. If you are underweight, the extra oxygen feeds the starving tissues and glands. In other words, yoga tends to produce the ideal weight for you.

8. Relaxation of the mind and body. Slow, deep, rhythmic breathing causes a reflex stimulation of the parasympathetic nervous system, which results in a reduction in the heart rate and relaxation of the muscles. These two factors cause a reflex relaxation of the mind, since the mind and body are very interdependent. In addition, oxygenation of the brain tends to normalize brain function, reducing excessive anxiety levels.

f. The breathing exercises cause an increase in the elasticity of the lungs and rib cage. This creates an increased breathing capacity all day, not just during the actual exercise period. This means all the above benefits also occur all day.

Section 17:
Posture

Foundation

Posture defines the health of your body as it aligns all the spinal segments and allows for a healthy nervous system and allows the Qi to flow through your body and the internal organs.

The key steps to proper posture both static and dynamic are:

70. Neutralize the pelvis and the hips

71. Core Activation and vertical elongation

72. Shoulder Balance

73. Neck retraction

74. Balanced Weight Bearing (no leaning to one side) both in standing and sitting.

Step 1: Neutralize Pelvis/ Hips

For many of us, our pelvis is tilted in such a way to cause weakness and dysfunction. This is mainly because we sit all or most of the day and spend hours with our legs bent. Also, we've habitually learned to "hang" on our bones rather than using our muscles to work for us, causing further weakening and dysfunctions.

Step II: Core Activation/ Vertical Elongation

Good posture starts with a strong core, which includes the deep transverse abdomens below the six pack, multifidus (deep low back muscles), diaphragm, and the pelvic floor. Strong core muscles don't just keep your back healthy and resistant to pain and injury; they also hold your body upright, improve balance and enable you to move your body with greater control and efficiency. If any (or all) of your core muscles are weak, other muscles have to compensate, resulting in the loss of motion, weakness, and pain. In fact, you can alleviate and prevent low back pain through regular core training.

Step III: Shoulder Balance

With increasing time spent in front of the computer, it's become more and more common to find people with forward shoulders (hunched shoulders and forward head). In these forward reaching positions, your chest, shoulders, and hip muscles become shortened and tight while the muscles of your upper and middle back weaken. You can improve your posture by strengthening the weak upper back muscles, while stretching tight muscles in the chest, shoulders, lats, and hips.

Step IV: Neck Retraction

Ideally, when viewed from the side, your ears should be above your shoulders. However, most people's heads (and therefore ears) push forward of the shoulders; this is usually accompanied by a protruding chin and rounded shoulders. This causes muscle imbalance and faulty postural habits that can cause long term problems. By fixing the tight and weak areas of the neck, your head will once again center itself just above the shoulders, if you had neck pain, this will fix this problem once and for all.

Step V: Balanced Weight Bearing

When standing, be conscious of your weight bearing tendencies. Make sure that you carry weight evenly between the left and the right feet. Chances are that you tend to lean to once side, usually the same side. When sitting, avoid crossing your legs, pay attention to the way your sits bones are carrying the weight. Remain conscious and aware of your posture while at work to ensure proper alignment and avoid muscle imbalances and faulty postural patterns.

Section 18:
Physical Therapy Approved Posture

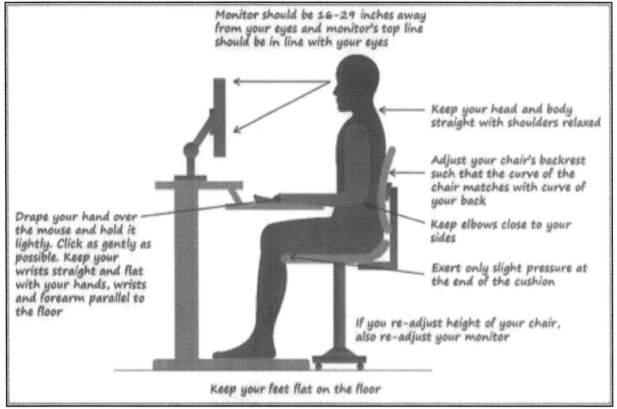

Proper Body Positioning at the work station

As a physical therapist, I see so many patients complaining of neck, shoulder, wrist, and back pain from prolonged sitting at the computers. With the work days averaging 8 hours a week, it's no wonder that more and more people are suffering from postural dysfunctions. Even when we come home, it's not uncommon for us to leisurely surf the web for various reasons.

Since it is impossible to eliminate the computers from our lives, let's look at some options and changes that we can make to ensure that we maintain healthy spines and decrease pain. Ergonomic Recommendations:

When possible, you should modify a computer workstation to best support a neutral body position. A Neutral body position is a comfortable working posture in which your joints are naturally aligned and there is the least stress and strain on your muscles, tendons, and joints. Sitting this way can help your tendons and joints heal. If you can, you should use a natural keyboard and sit in an ergonomic chair, which has an adjustable seat angle, back support, and padded elbow support. Here are some guidelines to help you maintain a neutral body position when sitting at a computer workstation.

Your hands, wrists, and forearms are straight, in-line and roughly parallel to the floor.

Your head is level, or bent slightly forward, forward facing, and balanced. Generally it is in-line with your torso.

Your shoulders are relaxed and upper arms hang normally at the side of the body.

Your elbows stay in close to the body and are bent between 90 and 120 degrees. Rest them on a padded elbow support if you have one on your chair

Your feet are fully supported on the floor.

Your back is fully supported with appropriate lumbar support when sitting vertical or leaning back slightly. Your low back and upper back are in neutral with a slight lordotic(extension) curve in your low back and a slight flexion in your Thoracic back. Neutral sitting is just relaxed from full extension and well away from a full slumped flexed posture. Your sternum is lifted slightly (sitting up and proud) and your shoulders are slightly back.

Your thighs and hips are supported by a well-padded seat and generally parallel to the floor.

Your knees are slightly lower than your hips with your feet slightly forward.

Regardless of how good your working posture is, working in the same posture or sitting still for prolonged periods is not healthy. Consider some of the following:

Stretch your fingers, hands, arms, and rotate your torso periodically.

Stand up periodically and stretch and walk around for a few minutes at your breaks.

Section 19:
The Alkaline Bath

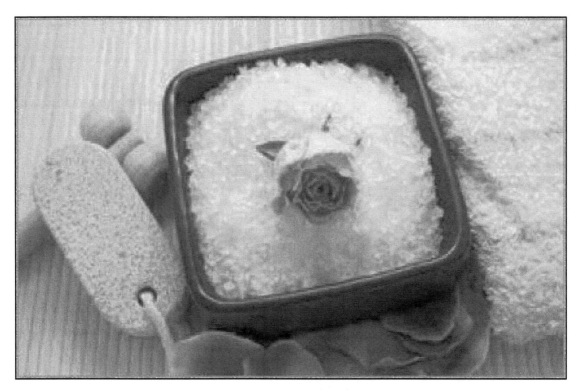

I've combined the benefits of the Epson bath with H-bath (Ultimate Fat Burning Bath) and have tried this for the last year with great success, I believe for the purpose of my program, the Ultimate 10 day Challenge, it will play a significant role in accelerating your efforts in healthy weight loss.

The Ultimate Fat Burning Bath has the following health benefits; relaxation inducing, improves circulation, detoxifying, increasing metabolism, promoting weight loss, increase energy, and pain alleviating.

Before I go any further, a little history of the baths..... The H-bath (Half Body Bath) was popularized in Korea and I was recommended to it by my oriental medicine/acupuncture doctor about a year ago. The h-bath was founded by Dr. Yoshiharu Shindo, who is a physician in Japan, and spread into Korea and China through the years. Epsom salts are made up of the compound magnesium sulfate, and they got their name because one of the earliest discoveries of magnesium and sulfate was in Epsom, England. The earliest use of salts and minerals for bathing was published in China around 2700 years BCE. Hippocrates also encouraged his fellow healers to make use of salt water to heal various ailments by immersing their patients in sea water. The ancient Greeks continued this, and in 1753 English author and physician Dr. Charles Russel published "The Uses of Sea Water" for humans for bathing for its healing capabilities.

For most of us, taking a bath means that we soak the whole-body (w-bath), which is submerging a body roughly the neck. In the early 1980's, Dr.Yoshiharu Shindo, a good ENT clinician, established some revolutionary bathing method, the actual half-body-bath (h-bath). Dr.Shindo mentions this in his primary book, [Remedy for all diseases - controlling the thermodynamics of the body];

A traditional w-bath (whole body bath) can produce lots of stress to the core, mainly caused by mineral water pressure. Since the whole is warmed up from the w-bath simultaneously the heart is enduring stress, the heart beat pace and blood pressure extremely fast increases and sometimes could potentially cause cardiac or vascular concerns. Besides, body heat can seldom be equilibrated since 85 - 90% of the body is submerged from the same temperature, and head is the only place to find the extreme blood stream as well as excess heat.

In contrast, the h-bath, the blood circulation accelerates gradually and reasonably with less stress in the heart. However, it doesn't suggest that the h-bath is "totally safe" for all populations, for elderly and coronary disease patients, you NEED to consult your doctor for medical clearance before starting the h-bath.

So why add Epson? Epson salt contains magnesium and magnesium is an essential element in the human body; it regulates enzymatic activity, it helps your internal organs function smoothly, and it keeps your skin soft as well.

I believe it is particularly beneficial to those of you in my program because the fact is that half of all Americans have a magnesium deficiency, which contributes to vast array of health problems according to the Epsom Salt Council. Soaking in the Epsom salt is beneficial because the magnesium can be absorbed through the skin. I recommend that you fill the bath tub 3-4 inches above your belly button (h-bath) and meditate and reflect for ultimate relaxation and stress relief as indicated in my program. Keep the water temperature as warm as you can handle (100-104 degrees) and soak in it no more than 20 minutes at a time. Again, I emphasize that you need to consult your medical doctor for health clearance prior to the bath.

You will sweat profusely during this process, keep in mind that all the sweat bubbles forming on your skin contains harmful toxins that has accumulated in your system. This is the main reason why I want all my clients to take regular h-baths in Epsom salt. The more you detoxify, improve functions of your internal organs, improve digestions, and ultimately improve metabolism. Toxins accumulated in your system causes inflammation and inflammation in your body causes weight gain. The toxins usually accumulate in your fat cells, you'll note that there are some legitimate claims for decreasing cellulite.

Proper way to take a Ultimate Bath:

1. Consider your tub size before you begin measuring the salt, more salt is not necessarily better. I recommend 1 -2 cups of Epsom salt to bath water that will soak you up to 3-4 inches above belly button when laying in the tub.

2. Temperature: I like to profusely sweat in my soaks, more sweat, more toxins out of me. However, make sure you use the temperature that is right for you. Safe effective range should be (100-104 degrees) which is slightly higher than your body temperature.

As beneficial as the H-Body Epson bath is, it is not for everyone. If you have heart problems, high blood pressure, or diabetes, please consult your doctor first.

3. Have a cold cup of water next to you and drink plenty of water to ensure that you are hydrated.

Where to purchase Epsom salt?

You can purchase Epsom salt at most grocery and health stores. I recently found a great product called "Dead Sea Magic Mineral" Bath Salts I found at the Whole Foods locally. I like it because it has various minerals in addition to the Magnesium. This is what I personally use, and I've been very pleased. You can go to their website; www.DeadSeaWarehouse.com

So soak up and enjoy...........it's extremely beneficial and effective as a regular regimen to lose weight and take control over your health.

Section 20:
Low Back Pain

It is estimated that about 80% to 90% of U.S. adults get low back pain at some point in their lives. Men and women are equally affected. Low back pain is more common as we get older, with people often having their first episode between ages 30 and 50. But it also can be the result of a sedentary lifestyle -- with too little (and occasionally too much) exercise. This puts most of the Americans at risk for low back pain. In the 12 years of clinical practice as physical therapist, low back pain is by far the most common diagnose for my patient base. Often, the pain can be debilitating and the pain is so severe that the patients often end up in the emergency.

Most of the patients want to know the culprit and try to replay the events leading up to the onset of symptoms. However, growing evidence proves that it is not an isolated event that caused the pain but cumulative effects of wear and tear over time. Take home lesson? Take good care of your back, especially your spine as we don't come with two sets.

Since low back pain is the fifth most common reason for doctor visits and the common immediate remedy is pain medications, anti-inflammatories, and possibly corticosteroid shots to the spine, many of my patients have figured out that the long term solution is to work at resolving the culprit of the issue, not masking the symptoms with the medications and the corticosteroid injections.

Please keep in mind that bed rest alone can actually make back pain worse. It can also lead to other conditions, like weakened muscles and blood clots in the legs. Remember my section on the Qi energy flow through the meridians. Low back pain can really block the essential energy channels resulting in a systemic condition that can be far worse than just low back pain. One study showed that patients who continued their normal activities after a bout of low back pain had more flexibility than those who rested in bed for a week. Staying in the same position for too long can also make your joints stiff and your Qi to be stagnant making the condition worse.

The lower back consists of five lumbar vertebrae. They are the weight-bearing part of the back and receive the most stress. The mid back is made up of 12 thoracic vertebrae. The ribcage attaches here. This part of the back is very flexible to allow bending and twisting. The seven cervical vertebrae are located in the neck. The spine should not be viewed as parts and pieces of the various sections, rather, it should be treated as a whole. Remember, your body is the sum of all its parts, everything works in synergy as one system.

Most back pain is caused by injury to the lower back or an ongoing condition. Overuse of the back muscles, sports injuries, extreme lifting, or sudden jolts -- such as a car accident -- are examples of injury. Arthritis or a bulging disc are ongoing conditions that may cause back pain.

Acute – or short-term – low back pain begins suddenly and may last several days or weeks. Chronic low back pain, which can be mild or severe, lasts longer than three months.

After the first flare-up, you might take a short rest period -- one to two days -- applying ice for the first couple of days and then a heating pad to loosen tight muscles. Take an over-the-counter pain medication if you need it just to keep the edge off the pain. You should try to stay active as much as possible. If you do choose a day of bed rest, try to walk around every couple of hours and schedule an appointment with an experienced physical therapist. Movement can help speed up healing, the sooner you can circulate the Qi energy the better. You should see your health care provider if the pain doesn't improve or if it gets worse within seven to 10 days.

As for the sleeping surfaces, firmer may not always be better. People who sleep on a medium-firm mattress are twice as likely to report that their back pain decreased while lying in bed or getting in or out of bed. So if you think you prefer a firm mattress, you might want to try medium-firm. Softer mattresses may place less pressure on the shoulders and hips, allowing you to sleep in a more natural position on your side. Your mattress should be firm enough to maintain your spine in the position you have with good standing posture.

Things like chiropractic care, physical therapy, yoga, and massage may help. In fact, groups such as the American Pain Society and American College of Physicians recommend these complementary and alternative treatments for people whose pain continues after more than a few weeks of self-care.

You should see a health care provider for back pain if you have any of the above symptoms or fever, weakness, trouble urinating, numbness in your legs, or weight loss when not on a diet. Most short-term low back pain is treatable without surgery, but these other symptoms may point to a more serious problem.

Remember, the more centralized your pain is the better. If you have radiating pain down the buttocks, thigh, legs into the feet, you are likely experiencing radiculopathy. Check with your physician first to make sure and have peace that physical therapy care can reverse the symptoms in due time. I advocate a functional approach to care where the patient takes responsibilities in their own care. I find that the more the patient is active in their own care, the better the outcome. Remember, we are prewired to have perfect health, we don't need others to snap us back or keep taking medications that get us further from our healing abilities.

Please remember that fewer than 2% of people with back pain have a herniated or slipped disk -- a bulging disk that presses on the nerves next to it. Most people with low back pain improve with treatment of heat and ice, rest, gentle exercise, and temporary over-the-counter pain relievers.

So remember, keep moving, consciously. I find that the more one gets out of touch with their body, the harder for our internal system to heal. You too will eventually heal, please be empowered

Part III:
Alkaline Diet

Genesis 1:29 ESV

And God said, "Behold, I have given you every plant yielding seed that is on the face of all the earth, and every tree with seed in its fruit. You shall have them for food.

 The concepts of the Alkaline Dieting is based on the eastern concept of cultivating health and longevity by balancing your unique energy with the universal energy. In other words, becoming aware of your universal environment and how the energetic forces can affect our own internal energy. The Qi energy is considered the circulating life energy, which is revered as the force that gives life to all things. Even foods have Qi energy and the art is in "balancing" these energy that you are eating to find optimal harmony.

In the human body, Qi flows through the energy pathways, referred to as the meridians. Meridians form an energy network that connects all organ systems in the body. And since this network of energy links all systems in the body, blockages in the meridians can cause significant problems in the body.

The meridians are sensitive to the changes of the environment. They have an inherent ability to keep the body in harmony. However, in the east, it is thought that the excess or deficiency of this energy can cause the body to be in a state of dis-ease. It is also understood that the foods can balance the excessive or deficient energy through proper activation of energy to various systems in the body.

What is a balanced meal?

The alkaline dieting will attempt to design a harmonious balance of all energies on a given meal. These energies include color, taste, texture, flavor, and shapes of food. The traditional cultures intuitively knew to eat according to climate and seasons. It is my ultimate goal to guide you in finding your intuition by listening to your body and its needs.

After working with numerous patients and clients, I found that many people have a difficult time changing their ways of eating. Eating is a ritual that is emotionally charged for most of us, we find comfort in the foods that nourished us while growing up for example. I for one had a personal experience with this as I knew that I needed to change my ways of eating as my digestive problems worsened. Even with the vast knowledge, it was very difficult for me. However, once you take the step in the right direction, you will find that it gets easier. As you go through the program, I encourage you to find your own relationship with food both the old and cultivate the new. I believe small changes over time become the very change that you want. It is human nature to want drastic changes in a short amount of time and it is important to realize that for those of us who wants to change our habits, we need to master our mind, not our conscious mind, but the sub-conscious. You see our sub-conscious mind drives approximately 90-95% of our behaviors. This is why we tend to continue with our habitual patterns even though we clearly know that it may not be the best for us. This is where also the concept of dieting fails because unless we "rewire" or "reprogram" our sub-conscious mind, we will revert back to our habits in due time. It is possible to make the changes that I am recommending and make it be an effortless process. I recommend that you read the chapter on the Alkaline Mind. For now, let me define the concept of Kaizen.

Kaizen was created in Japan following World War II. The word Kaizen means "continuous improvement". It comes from the Japanese words 改 ("kai") which means "change" or "to correct" and 善 ("zen") which means "good".

Although used mainly for businesses and productivity improvement, I want to introduce the concept here. Kaizen also implies small changes over time. The human mind is protective by nature, especially when you try to change a certain belief or behavior, you will have resistance. If you get discouraged for whatever reason, I want you to lay all things aside and take small steps every day. We usually want to make drastic changes but become very ineffective over time because drastic changes in behavior need the changes in the mind as well. In order to be more effective long term, please take it one step at a time. This hits home to me personally because I am an all or none type of person. In my mind, I feel I have to make drastic changes to make a huge difference. It's like the Hair and the Turtle story. In order to win this game, you need to be the turtle.

Once upon a time there was a hare who, boasting how he could run faster than anyone else, was forever teasing tortoise for its slowness. Then one day, the irate tortoise answered back: "Who do you think you are? There's no denying you're swift, but even you can be beaten!" The hare squealed with laughter.

"Beaten in a race? By whom? Not you, surely! I bet there's nobody in the world that can win against me, I'm so speedy. Now, why don't you try?"

Annoyed by such bragging, the tortoise accepted the challenge. A course was planned, and the next day at dawn they stood at the starting line. The hare yawned sleepily as the meek tortoise trudged slowly off. When the hare saw how painfully slow his rival was, he decided, half asleep on his feet, to have a quick nap. "Take your time!" he said. "I'll have forty winks and catch up with you in a minute."

The hare woke with a start from a fitful sleep and gazed round, looking for the tortoise. But the creature was only a short distance away, having barely covered a third of the course. Breathing a sigh of relief, the hare decided he might as well have breakfast too, and off he went to munch some cabbages he had noticed in a nearby field. But the heavy meal and the hot sun made his eyelids droop. With a careless glance at the tortoise, now halfway along the course, he decided to have another snooze before flashing past the winning post. And smiling at the thought of the look on the tortoise's face when it saw the hare speed by, he fell fast asleep and was soon snoring happily. The sun started to sink, below the horizon, and the tortoise, who had been plodding towards the winning post since morning, was scarcely a yard from the finish. At that very point, the hare woke with a jolt. He could see the tortoise a speck in the distance and away he dashed. He leapt and bounded at a great rate, his tongue lolling, and gasping for breath. Just a little more and he'd be first at the finish. But the hare's last leap was just too late, for the tortoise had beaten him to the winning post. Poor hare! Tired and in disgrace, he slumped down beside the tortoise who was silently smiling at him.

"Slow and steady does it every time!" he said.

Alkaline Dieting Fundamentals

1. Water is the most important in maintaining balance in the body.

We need to stay well hydrated at all times, after all, the human body is 70% water. Dehydration can have multiple adverse effects in our body; pain, illness, fatigue, and weight gain. When the body is dehydrated, the amount of lactic acid and metabolic acids increases, and toxins increase because the body's ability to "buffer" the acids and "detoxify" toxins become compromised. So remember, drink lots of water, also, those of you who have memory problems, this would be good reason, our brains are prone to dehydration.

2. Food Combining

There is a difference between alkaline foods and alkalizing foods. Important thing to remember is that the vegetables are generally alkalizing, meat protein sources are acidifying, fruits tend to be acidifying, and grains can go either way (more later). There is a way to combine the foods so that you optimize the alkalizing effects in the body. I won't go into it in detail but as a rule of thumb, keep the ratio of alkaline/acid foods to 70/30, (70 alkalizing and 30 acidic). -- Refer to the Alkaline Food Chart

3. Seasonal Foods

One thing that I want to emphasize is that we want to stay close to the laws of nature. God created the world and all organisms and we have natural order that was established. With the industrial revolution, we can now get vegetables, fruits, and grains from every part of the world, at any time of the year. However, it is best to eat seasonal foods, we have the energy force of the universe that have yin-yang characteristics and we want to make sure that summer time we eat more expansive yin fruits and vegetables, and in the winter, more contracted yang fruits and vegetables.

The way we cook is different for seasons, for example, in the winter, we tend to eat more stews, soups, hot teas and during the summer, we eat more of cold shakes, drinks, and dishes that require very little cooking. This tendency is the natural order, however, with the modern American Lifestyle, we pay very little attention to the natural wonders, such as the trees, birds, air, and general natural environments. Rather, we are usually surrounded by toxic environments and surroundings such as heaters, air conditioning, office space with no windows staring into the computer screens.

Respecting the universal order in selecting food is a macrobiotic approach and it is a good rule of thumb to follow. You will find that it is a simple way to drastically improve your general health and wellness.

4. Replenish Alkaline foods

We make acids in the body as metabolites, however, we don't really make alkaline substrates. Our body knows to "buffer" by neutralizing metabolic acids in the way of bile and some minerals such as Calcium, Magnesium, Iron, K, and

Sodium. Take home point here is that it's in our best interest to replenish our bodies with alkalizing foods to help keep our bodies alkaline.

4. Go Organic/ NO GMO products

There are many pesticides in our vegetables and fruits today and it accumulates in our bodies. This is my soap box, the governmental agencies do not protect us, there have been many attempts to draw attention to the negative effects of the pesticides but the government has been ignoring all claims. (this is controversial) Stay safe, these toxins are linked to numerous disease and symptoms. All your vegetables should be organic, as much as possible.

I am going to note that all animal source proteins are highly acidic and you want to make sure you are combining appropriately.

Livestock and Eggs: They are fed GMO soy and other grains, by order of nature, they are supposed to be eating pasture. They are also injected with antibiotics and hormones to "plump" up for increased revenue. In some cases they end up so diseased due to the unsanitary conditions that exist in the factory farms, it gives me chills and stomach pains just thinking about this.   If you must eat meat and eggs, eat grass-fed, antibiotic and hormone free, cage free, labels.

5. Eggs/Cheese/Milk

You want to be combining if you want to consume but just as above, go for the organic if you choose to eat this.

6. Sugar and Sweeteners

Read the labels, pay attention to sugar content, do not have foods that contain excess sugar. It's typically listed under carbohydrates, avoid foods that contain more than 10 gas per label. Make sure that they are no artificial, which includes equal, sweet n low, and splenda (aspartame, saccharin, sucrolose, and all sugar alcohols).

Avoid sweetened beverages, especially carbonated soft drinks.

Use natural sweeteners like stevia, molasses, or honey.

Absolutely NO high fructose corn syrup! No exceptions! HFCS is corn syrup that is processed with enzymes to convert glucose into fructose. It's mainly used in processed foods, especially in soft drinks.

7. Fats

Not all fats are bad. Use organic coconut oil, organic ghee (clarified butter), and organic extra virgin olive oil as raw or light sautéing.

Fish oil, grape seed oil, cod liver oil, and flaxseed oil in the raw are great contents of omega 3.

Fats in avocados, raw nuts, seeds are excellent.

Avoid "roasted "nuts and seeds, the roasting process causes rancidity in the fats and contain free radicals, which are inflammatory and toxic.

Avoid hydrogenated, or partially hydrogenated oil. It's in all packaged, processed foods such as crackers, chips, pretzels, cereal bars, popcorn, snacks.

When snacking, snack on the nutrient dense and good for you foods such as raw nuts, nut butters, fruits, veggies, boiled eggs, or smaller version of your actual meal, pieces of chicken, salads, etc.

8. Grains/Bread/Beans

Bread: consume "sprouted" whole grain (Ezekial or Manna Bread sold at whole food stores in the freezer section)

9. Salt

Eliminate all table or refined salt

Avoid canned foods that contain much sodium

Use unrefined salt, sea salt is a good option.

When cooking, add salt last.

10. Alcohol and Coffee

Alcohol and Coffee are highly acidic, it's best to avoid. Try green or herbal tea.....

The Five R Alkaline Matrix

1. Recognize:

Take a brief look around you and especially take note of what you are feeding yourself every day. I recommend that you keep a journal for 3 days to really be aware of your patterns. If you don't know what the problem is, you can't fix it. Also, I recommend that you take note of what you think about daily, what kind of internal dialogue do you have with yourself throughout your day? See the patterns especially notice the trigger thoughts that cause you to reach for food...., comfort foods. You'll notice that these foods tend to be sweet and high in calories. How many times a day do you eat? What kinds of cravings? Take a note of the "patterns" that you have.

2. Remove:

Based on the information provided above, remove all refined foods, simple sugars, processed foods, animal proteins, milk, cheese, etc., soft drinks, any carbonated drinks, coffee, alcohol, additives, all conventional produce (fruits and vegetables), conventional meats, egg, and cheese. Remove sugar rich foods and yeast in foods.

3. Replenish/Reprogram

Eat alkaline foods and use food combining techniques to optimize alkalinity and minimize acidity. Provide probiotics, supplementation based on needs such as a multivitamin, vit D, Fish Oil (Omega 3), pH drops for water, drink lots of water to flush out the toxins, phytonutrients, flax, eat diet rich in organic vegetables and fruits, sprouted grains. Use non GMO tofu, raw nuts, fish in moderation, organic chicken.

4. Repeat/Reconnect

Follow the above regimen for at least 21 days, if you get off track, get right back on track, and remember always to eat mindfully.

5. Restore/Restart

Restart the process with the deeper phases of alkaline program.

Section 21:
The Ultimate Truths about Food

"Knowledge is Power"

Food is thy Medicine---Hippocrates

Ultimate Truths:

Truth is that the food supply is not what it used to be. Agriculture farming has become a mega-business because mega-corporations are involved in food production on a large scale. This is problem that involves our food that affects the entire chain of agriculture related businesses, including seed supply, agri-chemicals, food processing, machinery, storage, transport, distribution, marketing, advertising, and retail sales. This means that farming's become a bonafide business and it has to be profitable for the corporations so whatever it takes to increase the profit margins, so will be.

"Corporate farming" is a term often used synonymously with "agribusiness". This farming practice is a common one in the United States today. Critics argue that the ultimate goal of corporate farming is to vertically integrate the entire process of food production. The problem is their heavy use of pesticides and chemical fertilizers that are used in the soil as well as the crops. This enables the agribusinesses to optimize their use of the surface area of the farmable land. This agricultural intensification has been the response to population growth, producing more food on the same amount of land. The problem is that the nutrient value of the crops and the toxic levels that they contain due to pesticides and chemical fertilizers pose a threat to the health of our nation. When going to the supermarket, they are labeled "conventional".

What does this mean for us consumers? First know the facts and be an advocate for sustainable farming practices. There is a organic movement today that support community sustained agriculture (CSA), basically means that the consumers directly buy from the local farmers that have safe organic practices that utilize the old fashioned method of farming that is both environmentally and agriculturally friendly. This allows us to eat fresh from local produce cutting down the fuel and energy required to ship and transport the crops from another region. If you look up CSA, you should be able to find some local to you. I typically go to the farmers market locally and buy my produce directly from the farmer. This allows me to have a relationship with my food and I know that I am doing my part to save the environment and eat fresh organic produce.

As for our meats, it too is a mega-business. "Factory farming" involves large numbers of animals raised on limited land, which require large amounts of food, water, and medical inputs (required to keep the animals healthy in cramped and unhealthy conditions). This very large of confined indoor intensive livestock operations are quite common US farming practices. This creates further pollution and health issues for both the consumers, animals, and the environment. In order to increase supply of eggs for example, the chicken is given hormones and antibiotics that enables them to produce the eggs. This too is an unnatural process, not to mention the cruelty to the animals. These animals are kept in such impossible situations that they require heavy doses of antibiotics just to keep them from infections that put them at risk due to filthy living quarters. These livestock are also injected hormones to "fatten" them up to get more cost per pound, not to mention the cattle is fed corn or grain to fatten them up, the truth is that the cows are supposed to be fed grass by nature. These unnatural practices inevitably make us question the health of the livestock that is readily available today.

On a pleasant note, the local farmers also raise livestock the way they are supposed to be raised, fed grass, are pastured, without antibiotics and hormones.

Solution

An ideal option would be to join a CSA (community sustained agriculture) and eat only the produce that grows locally.

Visit the farmers market regularly and buy your fresh produce there.

You can purchase organic meats from the below:

www.greensburymarket.com

www.wildwoodfoods.com/Organic

www.organicprairie.com/

www.localharvest.org/

Shop "organic" whenever possible at the local supermarkets.

Only eat seasonal produce.

Healthy Population and their secrets

SDA- Seventh Day Adventist

I am a proud graduate of Loma Linda University, I studied both Public Health Nutrition and Physical Therapy. During my studies, I was exposed to the very lifestyle factors of Seventh Day Adventist tradition that includes daily physical activity, observing Sabbath on Saturdays, no stimulants like black pepper, coffee, alcohol, no smoking, diet full of fresh vegetables and grains and little or no meat.

There is a study that involves the SDA population, called "Adventist Health Studies". This studied the long-term studies exploring the links between lifestyle, diet, and disease among Seventh-day Adventists. More than 96,000 church members from the U.S. and Canada are participating in the current study, AHS-2, conducted by researchers at the Loma Linda University School of Public Health.

Dietary Status of Study Members:

8% are vegan (No red meat, fish, poultry, dairy or eggs)

- 28% are lacto-ovo vegetarian (Consume milk and/or eggs, but no red meat, fish or poultry)

- 10% are pesco-vegetarian (Eat fish, milk and eggs but no red meat or poultry)

- 6% are semi-vegetarian (Eat red meat, poultry and fish less than once per week)

- 48% are non-vegetarian (Eat red meat, poultry, fish, milk and eggs more than once a week)

Findings:

The data showed that people who ate meet weighed significantly more compared to the vegetarian individual. For instance, 55-year-old male and female vegans weigh about 30 pounds less than non-vegetarians of similar height. Additionally, levels of cholesterol, diabetes, high blood pressure, and the metabolic syndrome all had the same trend – the closer you are to being a vegetarian, the lower the health risk in these areas. In the case of type 2 diabetes, prevalence in vegans and lacto-ovo vegetarians was half that of non-vegetarians, even after controlling for socioeconomic and lifestyle factors.

Although the results do not prove causation, they do suggest that possibility, thus, it is interesting to examine the characteristics of vegans/vegetarians.

Compared to non-vegetarians, vegans/vegetarians:

Watched less television

- Slept more hours per night

- Consumed more fruits and vegetables

- Consumed less saturated fat

- Typically ate foods with a low glycemic index, such as beans, legumes and nuts

Something to think about...and consider your current habits and see if you can modify some behaviors. It's the habits that are so powerful to ultimately set us on the right track.

Japanese

Elderly Okinawans have among the lowest mortality rates in the world from a multitude of chronic diseases of aging and as a result enjoy not only what may be the world's longest life expectancy but the world's longest health expectancy. Centenarians, in particular, have a history of aging slowly and delaying or sometimes escaping the chronic diseases of aging including dementia, cardiovascular disease (coronary heart disease and stroke) and cancer. The goal of the Okinawa Centenarian Study is to uncover the genetic and lifestyle factors responsible for this remarkable successful aging phenomenon for the betterment of the health and lives of all people.

The Okinawa Centenarian Study (OCS)　is an ongoing population-based study of centenarians and other selected elderly, in the Japanese prefecture of Okinawa that began in 1975. Ages are validated through the koseki, the Japanese family registration system. At the baseline exam a full geriatric assessment is performed, including physical exam and activities of daily living. Since the onset of the OCS, limited information on the demographics of the entire centenarian population of Okinawa has been collected and full assessments of a sub-sample of 900-plus centenarians have been performed.

When Dr. Suzuki, the Principal Investigator of the OCS, first began his studies, he found an unusual number of centenarians to be in extraordinarily healthy shape. They were lean, youthful-looking, energetic, and had remarkably low rates of heart disease and cancer-even stomach cancer, which claimed many mainland Japanese. And they enjoyed the longest life expectancy in the world. By 1995, according to Japan Ministry of Health and Welfare life tables, Okinawan life expectancy had even surpassed the absolute limits of population life expectancy estimated by the Japan Population Research Institute and many biodemographers (see Fries JF. New England Journal of Medicine 1980;303:131-5).

As can be deduced from these descriptions of a typical meal, the traditional dietary pattern in Okinawa has the following characteristics:

1) High consumption of vegetables,

2) High consumption of legumes (mostly soy in origin),

3) Moderate consumption of fish products (especially in coastal areas),

4) Low consumption of meat and meat products,

5) Low consumption of dairy products,

6) Moderate alcohol consumption,

7) Low caloric intake,

8) Rich in omega-3 fats,

9) High monounsaturated-to-saturated-fat ratio, and

10) Emphasis on low-GI carbohydrates.

vs.

SAD (Standard American Diet)

If you were to list the factors that increase the risk of cancer, heart disease, stroke, intestinal disorders – just about any illness – the standard American diet has them all:

High in animal fats

High in unhealthy fats: saturated, hydrogenated

Low in fiber

High in processed foods

Low in complex carbohydrates

Low in plant-based foods

The striking fact is that cultures that eat the reverse of the standard American diet – low fat, high in complex carbohydrates, plant-based, and high in fiber – have a lower incidence of cancer and coronary artery disease (CAD). What's even more sad is that countries whose populations can afford to eat the healthiest disease-preventing foods don't. The United States has spent more money on cancer research than any country in the world, yet the American diet contributes to the very diseases we are spending money to prevent. This seems counter productive.

My point is to ensure we follow the healthy proven habits to increase and improve our longevity, vitality, clarity, and energy.

Ultimate Protein Source

Meats: Grass fed, pastured meat contains muscle building blocks that are essential to our body. Grass fed beef contain more beta carotene, vitamin E, and omega 3 fatty acids than the conventional meats. They also have less fat per serving, than their conventional kind.

Fish: Wild caught fish, not ("farm" raised) also has high omega 3 content which is beneficial due to its anti-inflammatory effect in your body. The natural caught fish enables the fish to have the ideal composition that is desired. The mercury levels? Mercury levels are higher for tuna and swordfish, try to limit the intake of these.

What types of fish should you consume? Wild salmon, halibut, and cod are great choices that are full of the omega 3.

The omega 3's that are in these fish is important due to its effects on weight gain. The more you can reduce inflammation by consuming foods that are highly anti-inflammatory, like eating plenty of fish, veggies, and fruits, the easier it is for you to lose the fat and gain the lean muscle that you want.

Free Range, Organic Chicken : Have you noticed that when you buy the full rotisserie chicken, its bigger than ever before? I've wondered what are they feeding these chickens. Go with the free range, organic chicken. They not only taste better but contain more nutrients with ideal omega 3 to omega 6 ratio.

Organic Eggs: These are great sources of protein, especially the yolk, where the vitamins, minerals, and antioxidants are found. The yolk contains all of the fat soluble vitamins, A, D, E, and K as well as the essential fatty acids. Research has proven that the organic eggs contain 10X more omega 3 and are more nutrient rich than that of the conventional eggs.

Again, fresh eggs are usually available through the local farmer's market or CSA(Community Support Agriculture).

Nuts

Are nuts good for you and help you lose weight? Absolutely yes, take a handful a day as a healthy snack and take advantage of the high levels of vitamins and minerals. They are loaded with antioxidants and healthy fats that are actually great for your heart. But remember, nuts are highly caloric and are high in fat content, although good fat, be mindful and eat in moderation.

5 key Grains

Quinoa

While quinoa is usually considered to be a whole grain, it is actually a seed, but can be prepared like whole grains such as rice or barley. Try a quinoa in salads, or serve a vegetable stir fry over cooked quinoa instead of rice. Quinoa is my favorite whole grain for three reasons: First, it takes less time to cook than other whole grains – just 10 to 15 minutes. Second, quinoa tastes great on its own, unlike other grains such as millet or teff. Add a bit of olive oil, sea salt and lemon juice and - delicious! Finally, of all the whole grains, quinoa has the highest protein content, so it's perfect as a complete protein source especially if you are vegetarian or vegan. Quinoa provides all 9 essential amino acids, making it a complete protein. Quinoa is a gluten-free and cholesterol-free whole grain, is kosher, and is almost always organic.

Culinary experts will be interested to know that quinoa was a staple food for thousands of years in the Andes region of South America as one of just a few crops the ancient Incas cultivated at such high altitude.

Cooking quinoa:

Prepare quinoa as you would prepare rice. Cover it with water or vegetable broth and boil until soft, about 15 minutes. Or, place 1 part quinoa to 2 parts water in your rice cooker.

Barley

Whole grain barley is a healthy high-fiber, high-protein whole grain, boasting numerous health benefits. When cooked, barley has a chewy texture and nutty flavor, similar to brown rice. Although soup is the most common way to eat barley, you can use it like any other grain such as couscous or rice. Serve with curry or stir fry over barley instead of rice or make a barley pilaf. Barley is Chewy and nutty, it may be more widely enjoyed as an ingredient in beer than in its whole grain state, but that doesn't mean you shouldn't give it a try! Like many whole grains, barley has been shown to be effective in lowering cholesterol particularly in men. If you're looking to eat more whole grains to reduce your cholesterol, barley may be the best one to try. It'll really stick to your ribs and fill you up, too. Toasted barley is often used as a coffee substitute, but I like my barley in soup with plenty of mushrooms.

How to cook barley:

Cooking barley is similar to cooking rice. Cover 1 cup of pearl barley with 2 cups of water or vegetable broth and simmer for 30-40 minutes before fluffing with a fork. Or, try using a rice cooker. Add 2 1/2 cups water per cup of barley.

Bulgar Wheat

Bulgur wheat is a whole wheat grain that has been cracked and partially pre-cooked. As a whole grain, it is a naturally high-fiber, low-fat, low-calorie vegetarian and vegan appropriate. Bulgur wheat is not suitable for those on a gluten-free diet.

Cooking bulgur wheat

Though bulgur wheat is most commonly found in tabouli (tabbouleh) salad, you can use it just like rice or couscous, or any other whole grain, such as barley or quinoa. Instead of rice, try pairing your favorite stir-fry or curry with whole grain bulgur. Or, try one of the easy bulgur wheat recipes below.

Types of bulgur wheat

Different types of bulgur wheat require different cooking times, so its best to check the package instructions for cooking instructions. One advantage of using bulgur wheat is that is has already been partially cooked, so it can be quick and easy to prepare at home.

Instant bulgur, also called fine-grain bulgur is common in health food store bulk bins and is usually used for tabbouli recipes. This type of bulgur cooks in less than 5 minutes. Medium grain and coarse grain are also available.

Shopping for bulgur wheat

Nearly all health food stores stock bulgur wheat. Look in the bulk foods section, or in the baking aisle. If that doesn't work, check the cereal aisle, or ask the staff for assistance.

Nutritional value of bulgur wheat

According to calorie count, one cup of cooked bulgur wheat provides 151 calories, 0.4 grams of fat, 8.2 grams of dietary fiber (that's about 33% the recommended daily value), and a healthy 5.6 grams of protein. Bulgur wheat is naturally cholesterol-free food.

Buckwheat

Buckwheat, which is commonly found in raw food diet recipes, has a slightly deceptive name that can easily cause confusion. Buckwheat is not wheat, nor is it related to wheat. It is not a grain nor a cereal and is gluten-free. So where does it come from? Buckwheat is derived from the seeds of a flowering plant.

Culinary Uses of Buckwheat

The triangular seeds, known as buckwheat groats, are frequently made into flour for use in noodles, crepes, and many gluten-free products on the market these days. For those practicing a raw food diet, raw buckwheat groats can be found in many recipes for things like granola, cookies, cakes crackers, and other bread like products. Buckwheat is a good binding agent and, when soaked, becomes very gelatinous. Soaking, rinsing, and re-drying the groats produces a crunchy buckwheat crispy that is nice as well.

Raw Buckwheat and Kasha

Toasted buckwheat is used to make traditional dishes in several different cultures. Generally toasted buckwheat is referred to as kasha. If you are looking for raw buckwheat groats, you'll want to avoid kasha. You can always tell by the color and the aroma. Kasha is a much darker reddish-brown color and has a strong nutty, toasted scent to it. Raw buckwheat groats are light brown or green and don't have much of an aroma at all.

Nutritional Benefits of Buckwheat

Interestingly, buckwheat is currently being studied for its nutritional benefits. It is used to relieve some of the symptoms of Type II diabetes as well as high blood pressure. Buckwheat contains rutin, known to strengthen capillary walls. "about.com"

Wheat berries

Wheat berries are the whole grain form of wheat - the whole complete grain before it has undergone any processing. They're a high-fiber whole grain that can be used much like any other whole grain.

How to prepare wheat berries?

Wheat berries can be tough so keep in mind, whole grain wheat berries do take a long time to cook. To prepare wheat berries, cover them with plenty of water and simmer in a covered pot for about one hour, or until soft. Serve cooked wheat berries with a vegetable stir-fry or a sauce, or use it like you would use rice. For a quicker cooking time, wheat berries can be pre-soaked overnight, or even just for an hour or two.

Millets

The millets, a group of thousands of varieties of grass-like annual plants that bear small to miniscule-sized seeds belong to the Gramineae family of plants.

Millet is considered the 6th most important grain crop in the world.

The most common varieties of millet include pearl, proso, foxtail, finger and teff (Ethiopian millet). Millet has been a major source of protein and energy for millions of people in Asia, Africa and India for thousands of years.

Most of the millet grown in the US is used as birdseed and animal feed but millet and teff are highly nutritious, gluten-free whole grain and flour products.

Nutritional Benefits of Using Millet in Gluten-Free Cooking:

Millet contains high levels of two essential amino acids (proteins), methionine and cysteine. Our bodies need adequate supplies of all of the essential amino acids for growth and cellular repair. Most grains, including rice, corn, wheat and sorghum have low levels of these two important proteins. Millet, like wheat and corn is low in another essential amino acid, lysine. Millet is considered easier to digest than most grains.

Teff is a good source of iron, calcium, magnesium and zinc. Millet is a good source of fiber.

Ultimate Fat Source

Confused About Fats? The following nutrient-rich traditional fats have nourished healthy population groups for thousands of years:

For Cooking

Butter

Coconut, palm and palm kernel oils

Ghee

For Salads

Extra virgin olive oil (also OK for cooking)

Expeller-expressed sesame and peanut oils

Expeller-expressed flax oil (in small amounts)

For Fat-Soluble Vitamins

Fish liver oils such as cod liver oil (preferable to fish oils, which do not provide fat-soluble vitamins, can cause an overdose of unsaturated fatty acids and usually come from farmed fish.)

Note: The following newfangled fats can cause cancer, heart disease, immune system dysfunction, sterility, learning disabilities, growth problems and osteoporosis:

All hydrogenated and partially hydrogenated oils

Industrially processed liquid oils such as soy, corn, safflower, cottonseed and canola

Fats and oils (especially vegetable oils) heated to very high temperatures in processing and frying.

The Many Roles of Saturated Fat

Saturated fats (the "good" fats), such as butter, meat fats, coconut oil and palm oil, tend to be solid at room temperature. According to conventional nutritional dogma, these traditional fats are to blame for most of our modern diseases-- heart disease, cancer, obesity, diabetes, malfunction of cell membranes and even nervous disorders like multiple sclerosis.

However, many scientific studies indicate that it is processed liquid vegetable oil--which is laden with free radicals formed during processing--and artificially hardened vegetable oil--called trans fat--that are the culprits in these modern conditions, not natural saturated fats.

Humans need saturated fats because we are warm blooded. Our bodies do not function at room temperature, but at a tropical temperature. Saturated fats provide the appropriate stiffness and structure to our cell membranes and tissues. When we consume a lot of liquid unsaturated oils, our cell membranes do not have structural integrity to function properly, they become too "floppy," and when we consume a lot of trans fat, which is not as soft as saturated fats at body temperature, our cell membranes become too "stiff."

Contrary to the accepted view, which is not scientifically based, saturated fats do not clog arteries or cause heart disease. In fact, the preferred food for the heart is saturated fat; and saturated fats lower a substance called Lp(a), which is a very accurate marker for proneness to heart disease.

Saturated fats play many important roles in the body chemistry. They strengthen the immune system and are involved in inter-cellular communication, which means they protect us against cancer. They help the receptors on our cell membranes work properly, including receptors for insulin, thereby protecting us against diabetes.

The lungs cannot function without saturated fats, which is why children given butter and full-fat milk have much less asthma than children given reduced-fat milk and margarine. Saturated fats are also involved in kidney function and hormone production.

Saturated fats are required for the nervous system to function properly, and over half the fat in the brain is saturated. Saturated fats also help suppress inflammation. Finally, saturated animal fats carry the vital fat-soluble vitamins A, D and K2, which we need in large amounts to be healthy.

Human beings have been consuming saturated fats from animals products, milk products and the tropical oils for thousands of years; it is the advent of modern processed vegetable oil that is associated with the epidemic of modern degenerative disease, not the consumption of saturated fats.

by Sally Fallon Morell

Ultimate Truths about Sugar

The average American now consumes 175 pounds of sugar per year! That's 46 teaspoons a day!   But the truth is that sugar has absolutely no nutritional value whatsoever. Not only does it totally lack nutrients, but when you eat sugar it actually robs your body of nutrients-- vitamins, minerals and even enzymes.

The sad thing is that most people are not aware of the devastating effects that excess sugar consumption has on the body.   The following steps are necessary to change your sugar habits.

Step 1. Eliminate all sugar drinks

Avoid all sodas, powdered drinks, sports drinks and fruit juices (basically anything in a can, bottle or drink box). Instead, drink plenty of clean water (reverse osmosis filtration is best). It can be flavored with juice of lemon, orange, or essential oils like cinnamon, tangerine or peppermint. Also, herb teas make tasty drinks and come in many delicious flavors (but avoid those with added "flavorings"). Try serving tea chilled and add a pinch of stevia (a natural low-calorie sweetener available at health food stores). If you have access to some sour lacto-fermented drinks or are willing to make them, these would be great.

Step 2. Cut out the sugar habit

Once you have given up the habit of eating sweets on a daily basis, it is common to experience symptoms like nausea, headache, fatigue, or dizziness after indulging in sweets. After giving up sweets for a while, many people say that they don't even taste that good anymore.

Step 3. Make a habit of eating at least two good meals per day

One of the best ways to overcome cravings for sweets is to eat small frequent healthy meals and snacks to keep your blood sugar levels even. To build a balanced meal, begin with a protein, include a natural source of carbohydrates (veggies, legumes, properly prepared whole grains, or fruits), and don't forget the good fats (butter, coconut, oil, palm oil, avocados and olive oil). Don't be afraid to eat lots of good fat at every meal. Fats slow down the entry of sugar into the blood stream and prevent those morning and afternoon crashes. If your breakfast, lunch and dinner are filled with nutritious, high-fat foods, you probably won't even think about snack foods between meals.

Step 4. Replace refined sugars with natural sugars

Get in the habit of reading labels and avoid products made with white sugar, corn syrup, high fructose corn syrup, sucrose, dextrose, fructose, and ALL artificial sweeteners. Instead use natural sweeteners, including

pure maple syrup, molasses, stevia, Rapadura (dehydrated cane sugar juice) or raw unfiltered honey.

Many health food stores offer products made with natural sweeteners, like cookies and ice cream, and even licorice, although it is better to make your own. Use this step to help you become acquainted with all the natural alternatives to replace refined sugar products.

Step 5. Limit natural sweets to three times per week

Blood sugar imbalances occur after eating too many sweets, even the natural ones! So it's important to limit even the natural sweets in your diet. And remember, the best way to prevent sweets from causing a major crash in blood sugar is to avoid eating them by themselves. Instead include dessert as part of a balanced meal. A steak with some steamed veggies, a salad topped with olive oil-based dressing, and a couple of natural cookies made with butter and eggs would be a healthy and balanced way to include dessert.

Eliminating refined sugar can be quite a challenging step, but the incredible impact it will have on your overall health and well-being is definitely worth it! Be patient with yourself through this process. Many times people try to quit sugar "cold turkey," but end up dreaming about it all day long until eventually they binge on sweets. Then they are right back on the blood-sugar roller coaster. The goal is to stabilize your blood sugar by eating balanced meals at regular intervals throughout the day so that you no longer crave sweets. True success comes when you do eat sweets and they no longer taste good, better yet, they give you a headache, make you nauseous, tired, dizzy and depressed!

Ultimate Truths about Dairy

The biggest concern with today's' dairy is the use of antibiotics, pesticides, and hormones that are used on the cows. There's so much information out there regarding this topic, to drink/consume or not to drink/consume. I believe this article will shed some light on what is right for you.

There is significant evidence indicating that people who consume a diet that is rich in fruits and vegetables tend to be healthier than those who consume a diet that is rich in meat and processed food. I believe it is an individual choice to be a vegetarian or choose to consume meat, poultry, or fish. In either case, as long as the diet is full of unprocessed, whole foods in its natural state, its acceptable.

Is Milk Good for you?

It all depends on where it comes from, doesn't it?

The subject of milk sparks just about as much controversy as the subject of fats. Many alternative practitioners feel that it's not necessary for humans to consume cow's milk and link its consumption to health problems, such as ear infections, allergies, cancer and diabetes. On the other hand, the medical community has convinced us that if we don't drink enough milk our bones will disintegrate. And the American Dairy Association promotes milk by celebrity endorsements. So let's review the milk controversy.

Living Conditions

If I were to ask you to picture a cow, you would most likely see in your mind a cow grazing in an open pasture, like one you'd probably seen before on a small family farm. That's a lucky cow, compared to most of the cows bred for dairy production in this country. The majority of commercial dairy cows don't have the luxury of grazing on open fields. Picture them in intense confinement, in individual stalls, on hard cement floors, hooked up to milking machines, forced to produce milk ten months out of the year. This is how the average commercial dairy cow spends her short, miserable life--42 months on average, compared to 12-15 years for a cow on pasture. The fact is, this is not the way mother nature designed the milk production for them. They are supposed to be enjoying the pasture, feeding on grass with no stress hormones raging into their milk. Yes, the milk that we and our kids drink.

Environment

Not only is the unnatural building environment a problem for the cow, but it can be a huge problem for the people around it as well. The cows in this environment produce massive amount of waste and can have devastating effects on the surrounding environment. The truth is over one-fifth of the country's dairy products are produced in the central valley of California where confinement operations create as much waste as a city of 21 million people! Much of that waste is forced unnaturally into the environment, polluting our lakes, rivers and streams. Not very sustainable practice, goes against mother nature. On the flip side, small farms are able to recycle manure back into the earth to enrich the soil. This is where the ecosystem, the way God designed it can thrive.

Feed

A cow's natural diet consists mostly of grass, however, since there isn't enough grass or the field to go around on the factory farm, they are fed mostly grain, and other things that they would not normally eat. The bulk of the feed consists of corn and soy, which receives 80 percent of all herbicides used in the US. When we think of pesticides we usually think of produce, but animal products can contain up to 14 times more pesticides than plants!1

Simply switching the cow's diet from grass to grain can cause many problems, but that's only the beginning. According to a recent article in US News & World Report, some 40 billion pounds a year of slaughterhouse wastes like blood, bone and viscera, as well as the remains of millions of euthanized cats and dogs passed along by veterinarians and animal shelters, are rendered annually into livestock feed, shocking!

That's not all, the animal-feed manufacturers and farmers also have begun using dehydrated food garbage, fats emptied from restaurant fryers and grease traps, cement-kiln dust, in some cases, newspapers and cardboard that are derived from plant cellulose.

During the BSE scare, the FDA ordered a halt to feeding all slaughterhouse wastes to cattle and sheep in the US. At that time 75 percent of the nation's 90 million cattle had been eating feed containing slaughterhouse by-products!

Like humans, animals need nutrients to thrive and be healthy. It is obvious that the factory farm houses do not supply the cows with the proper nourishment. Instead, they are only interested in stuffing whatever they can into the cows to fatten them up as quickly as possible. This leads to sick livestock and the solution is in injecting antibiotics and medications that further pollute the milk. Like pesticides, these drugs end up in the milk of the dairy animals, as do trans fats from bakery wastes, undigested proteins from soy and animal foods and aflatoxins from moldy grain. What's worse is that these byproducts are highly concentrated in the milk.

Antibiotics

Did you know that if you drink commercial milk or eat commercially raised meats and poultry, you could be consuming antibiotics on a daily basis without even knowing it! Over 50 percent of all the antibiotics produced in this country are mixed directly into animal feed. Ideally, antibiotics should be used in farming only when necessary to treat infection. However, due to the sickly nature of factory farmed animals, they are fed a constant supply of antibiotics from birth until the time of slaughter.

Antibiotic resistance is a serious issue that has gotten a lot of press in recent years. Basically, bacteria are mutating and outsmarting the antibiotics, making them ineffective. (The same phenomenon is occurring on farms where bugs are mutating to withstand pesticide applications.) We criticize medical doctors for over-prescribing antibiotics, but that is only part of the problem. Not only are antibiotics overused in this country, but they are also over-consumed. People are unknowingly consuming more antibiotics than they are actually taking by choice. Due to the heavy doses of antibiotics used on factory farmed animals, your steaks, hamburgers, chicken, and hotdogs are all contain antibiotics.

Hormones

CAPTION: A typical modern dairy cow. Her udder is so full it almost drags on the ground and she must be milked three times per day. Note the unusual growth in front of her forelegs--a goiter or a tumor?

Historically, in 1930, the average dairy cow produced 12 pounds (about a gallon and a half) of milk per day. In 1988, the average was increased to 39 pounds per day. This was accomplished by selective breeding to obtain dairy cows that produced a lot of pituitary hormones, thereby generating large amounts of milk. But the industry was not satisfied with this output, they wanted more. Today rBGH, a synthetic growth hormone, is used to get even more milk out of the dairy cows, bringing the average up to 50 pounds (over 6 gallons) of milk per day, astounding!

When you mess with mother nature, the outcome is not only scary but also unknown. It is reported that the cows injected with rBGH is more likely to suffer from mastitis. Other problems can include reproductive difficulties, increased need for antibiotics, digestive problems, enlarged hocks and lesions, and foot problems.

According to the Humane Farming Association, The FDA admits that BGH injections increase sickness and drug use in dairy cows. Consumers Union reports that because of increased udder infections, it is more likely that milk from treated cows will be of lower quality--containing more pus and bacteria-- than milk from untreated cows.

Pasteurization

Pasteurization is a process of heat treating milk to kill bacteria. This was developed by Louis Pasteur to preserve beer and wine; however, he was not responsible for applying it to milk. That was done at the end of the 1800s as a temporary solution until filthy urban dairies could find a way to produce cleaner milk. But instead of cleaning up milk production, dairies used pasteurization as a way to cover up dirty milk. As milk became more mass produced, pasteurization became necessary for large dairies to increase their profits. So the public then had to be convinced that pasteurized milk was safer than raw milk. Soon raw milk consumption was blamed for all sorts of diseases and outbreaks until the public was finally convinced that pasteurized milk was superior to milk in its natural state.

Today if you mention raw milk, many people gasp and utter ridiculous statements like, "You can die from drinking raw milk!" But the truth is that there are far more risks from drinking pasteurized milk than unpasteurized milk. Raw milk naturally contains healthy bacteria that inhibit the growth of undesirable and dangerous organisms. Without these friendly bacteria, pasteurized milk is more susceptible to contamination. Furthermore, modern equipment, such as milking machines, stainless steel tanks and refrigerated trucks, make it entirely possible to bring clean, raw milk to the market anywhere in the US.

Not only does pasteurization kill the friendly bacteria, it also greatly diminishes the nutrient content of the milk. Pasteurized milk has up to a 66 percent loss of vitamins A, D and E. Vitamin C loss usually exceeds 50 percent. Heat affects water soluble vitamins and can make them 38 percent to 80 percent less effective. Vitamins B6 and B12 are completely destroyed during pasteurization. Pasteurization also destroys beneficial enzymes, antibodies and hormones. Pasteurization destroys lipase (an enzyme that breaks down fat), which impairs fat metabolism and the ability to properly absorb fat soluble vitamins A and D. (The dairy industry is aware of the diminished vitamin D content in commercial milk, so they fortify it with a form of this vitamin.)

We have all been led to believe that milk is a wonderful source of calcium, when in fact, pasteurization makes calcium and other minerals less available. Complete destruction of phosphatase is one method of testing to see if milk has been adequately pasteurized. Phosphatase is essential for the absorption of calcium.

Homogenization

Raw milk straight from the cow contains cream, which rises to the top. Homogenization is a process that breaks up the fat globules and evenly distributes them throughout the milk so that they do not rise. This process unnaturally increases the surface area of fat exposing it to air, in which oxidation occurs and increases the susceptibility to spoilage. Homogenization has been linked to heart disease and atherosclerosis. Again, ignoring mother nature presents with dire consequences.

Milk: To Drink or Not to Drink?

It's no wonder that millions of Americans are allergic to the commercial, pasteurized milk. An allergic reaction to dairy can cause symptoms like diarrhea, vomiting (even projectile vomiting), stomach pain, cramping, gas, bloating, nausea, headaches, sinus and chest congestion, and a sore, or scratchy throat. Milk consumption has been linked to many other health conditions as well, such as asthma, atherosclerosis, diabetes, chronic infections (especially upper respiratory and ear infections), obesity, osteoporosis and cancer of the prostate, ovaries, breast and colon.

However, real, raw Milk--full-fat, unprocessed milk from pasture-fed cows-- contains vital nutrients like fat-soluble vitamins A and D, calcium, vitamin B6, B12, and CLA (conjugated linoleic acid, a fatty acid naturally occurring in grass-fed beef and milk that reduces body fat and protects against cancer). Real milk is a source of complete protein and is loaded with enzymes. Raw milk contains beneficial bacteria that protects against pathogens and contributes to a healthy flora in the intestines. Culturing milk greatly enhances its probiotic and enzyme content, making it a therapeutic food for our digestive system and overall health.

I do recommend that you drink milk if you can get it from a local farmer who offer the "raw" milk.

REFERENCES

Nutrition News and Views, Nov/Dec 1999, Vol 3, No.6, p. 2.

The Next Bad Beef Scandal?" US News & World Report, September 1, 1997.

Nutrition News and Views, Nov/Dec 1999, Vol 3, No.6, p 2.

Mark Kastel, Down on the Farm: The Real BGH Story- Animal Health Problems, Financial Troubles," published by Rural Vermont, 1991.

Andrew Christiansen, Recombinant Bovine Growth Hormone: Alarming Tests, Unfounded Approval: The Story Behind the Rush to Bring rBGH to Market," published by Rural Vermont, 1991.

Ultimate Truths about Soy

SOY DANGERS SUMMARIZED

- High levels of phytic acid in soy reduce assimilation of calcium, magnesium, copper, iron and zinc.

- Phytic acid in soy is not neutralized by ordinary preparation methods such as soaking, sprouting and long, slow cooking, but only with long fermentation.

- High phytate diets have caused growth problems in children.

- Trypsin inhibitors in soy interfere with protein digestion and may cause pancreatic disorders.

- In test animals, soy containing trypsin inhibitors caused stunted growth.

- Soy phytoestrogens disrupt endocrine function and have the potential to cause infertility and to promote breast cancer in adult women.

- Soy phytoestrogens are potent antithyroid agents that cause hypothyroidism and may cause thyroid cancer. In infants, consumption of soy formula has been linked to autoimmune thyroid disease.

- Vitamin B12 analogs in soy are not absorbed and actually increase the body's requirement for B12.

- Soy foods increase the body's requirement for vitamin D. Toxic synthetic vitamin D2 is added to soy milk.

- Fragile proteins are over-denatured during high temperature processing to make soy protein isolate and textured vegetable protein.

- Processing of soy protein results in the formation of toxic lysinoalanine and highly carcinogenic nitrosamines.

- Free glutamic acid or MSG, a potent neurotoxin, is formed during soy food processing and additional amounts are added to many soy foods to mask soy's unpleasant taste.

- Soy foods contain high levels of aluminum, which is toxic to the nervous system and the kidneys.

- Lastly, there is a lot of controversy about the GMO (genetically modified organism), crops may threaten biodiversity, decrease the richness and variety of foods, and make farmers more dependent on chemical companies, through the purchase of seed or chemicals.

- Health concerns include: allergy, gene transfer (antibiotic-resistant genes from GMO to bacteria), and out crossing (the movement of genes from GMO plants into conventional crops).

Conclusion, avoid soy products when you can, especially the GMO kind. The above list is the proof, need I say more?

Read your labels!

Ultimate Hydration

How much water should you drink each day? Studied have produced varying recommendations over the years, but in truth, your water requirement depends on various factors such as your health, how active you are, and where you live.

How much water do you need?

Every day you lose water through your breath, perspiration, urine and bowel movements. For your body to function properly, you must replenish its water supply by consuming beverages and foods that contain water.

So how much fluid does the average, healthy adult living in a temperate climate need? The Institute of Medicine determined that an adequate intake (AI) for men is roughly 3 liters (about 13 cups) of total beverages a day. The AI for women is 2.2 liters (about 9 cups) of total beverages a day.

What about the advice to drink eight glasses a day?

Everyone has heard the advice, "Drink eight 8-ounce glasses of water a day." That's about 1.9 liters, which isn't that different from the Institute of Medicine recommendations. Although the "8 by 8" rule isn't supported by hard evidence, it remains popular because it's easy to remember. Just keep in mind that the rule should be reframed as: "Drink at least eight 8-ounce glasses of fluid a day," because all fluids count toward the daily total.

Factors that affect water needs:

You may need to modify your total fluid intake depending on how active you are, the climate you live in, your health status, and if you're pregnant or breast-feeding.

Exercise.

If you exercise or engage in any activity that makes you sweat, you need to drink extra water to compensate for the fluid loss. An extra 400 to 600 milliliters (about 1.5 to 2.5 cups) of water should suffice for short bouts of exercise, but intense exercise lasting more than an hour (for example, running a marathon) requires more fluid intake. How much additional fluid you need depends on how much you sweat during exercise, and the duration and type of exercise. During long bouts of intense exercise, it's best to use a sports drink that contains sodium, as this will help replace sodium lost in sweat and reduce the chances of developing hyponatremia, which can be life-threatening. Also, continue to replace fluids after you're finished exercising. I especially like the coconut water because it also contains the alkalizing minerals such as magnesium that you lost through your sweat.

Climate

Hot or humid weather can make you sweat and requires additional intake of fluid. Heated indoor air also can cause your skin to lose moisture during wintertime. Further, altitudes greater than 8,200 feet (2,500 meters) may trigger increased urination and more rapid breathing, which use up more of your fluid reserves.

Illnesses or health conditions.

When you have fever, vomiting or diarrhea, your body loses additional fluids. In these cases, you should drink more water. In some cases, your doctor may recommend oral rehydration solutions, such as Gatorade, Powerade or CeraLyte. However, remember that these drinks also contain additives, coloring, and in most cases, high fructose corn syrup, so instead, reach for coconut water. Also, you may need increased fluid intake if you develop certain conditions, including bladder infections or urinary tract stones. On the other hand, some conditions such as heart failure and some types of kidney, liver and adrenal diseases may impair excretion of water and even require that you limit your fluid intake.

Pregnancy or breast-feeding. Women who are expecting or breast-feeding need additional fluids to stay hydrated. Large amounts of fluid are used especially when nursing. The Institute of Medicine recommends that pregnant women drink 2.3 liters (about 10 cups) of fluids daily and women who breast-feed consume 3.1 liters (about 13 cups) of fluids a day.

Beyond the H2O, Other sources of water

Although it's a great idea to keep water within reach at all times, you don't need to rely only on what you drink to meet your fluid needs. What you eat also provides a significant portion of your fluid needs. On average, food provides about 20 percent of total water intake. For example, many fruits and vegetables, such as watermelon and tomatoes, are 90 percent or more water by weight.

In addition, beverages such as milk and juice are composed mostly of water. Water is still your best bet because it's calorie-free, inexpensive and readily available. Highly recommend filtered water.

Staying safely hydrated

Generally if you drink enough fluid so that you rarely feel thirsty and produce 1.5 liters (6.3 cups) or more of colorless or light yellow urine a day, your fluid intake is probably adequate. If you're concerned about your fluid intake or have health issues, check with your doctor or a registered dietitian. He or she can help you determine the amount of water that's right for you.

To ward off dehydration and make sure your body has the fluids it needs, make water your beverage of choice.

Drink water before, during and after exercise.

Although uncommon, it is possible to drink too much water. When your kidneys are unable to excrete the excess water, the electrolyte (mineral) content of the blood is diluted, resulting in low sodium levels in the blood, a condition called hyponatremia. However, unless you are an endurance athlete, such as marathon runners, who drink large amounts of water, no need to worry. In general, though, drinking too much water is rare in healthy adults who eat an average American diet.

Ultimate position on Coffee Vs. Tea

That delicious fragrant morning brew that wakes us up every morning….how can this be so bad? I think drinking coffee is a ritual for many who don't want to give up than the coffee itself. So is this "coffee"……..is it so bad for you, especially when it comes to losing weight? I think you should make an informed choice, I say this because unless it's something that will kill me, I was not ready to give up coffee, I love coffee that much. I haven't figured out if it's the "ritual" that my subconscious is refusing to give up or it's the actual caffeine that I need.

I want to put things in perspective for you, it's not the coffee, and it's the caffeine in the coffee. It's also the extras that coffees come with, such as cream, milk, in latte's, caramel, and chocolate in macchiato. Often people think of coffee just as a vehicle for caffeine. But it's actually a very complex beverage with hundreds and hundreds of different compounds in it. Since coffee contains so many different compounds, drinking coffee can lead to very diverse health outcomes. Coffee is in the very fiber of an American life, it seems you can't drive a mile without a Starbucks these days.

Five minutes after you've downed that morning Java, the caffeine begins to stimulate your central nervous system, releasing stress hormones and creating an internal emergency response. If you're facing a life-threatening situation, this can be useful, but if you're at a desk, playing with your kid or reading a paper, you may begin feeling agitated, anxious, hungry and eventually exhausted. In this condition, you're usually temped to eat more sweet food or take more coffee…and the cycle continues until burn-out.

Equally important is that caffeine stimulates the production of norepinephrine, another stress hormone that acts directly on the brain and nervous system. Epinephrine and norepinephrine are two hormones responsible for increased heart rate, elevated blood pressure, and that "emergency response" feeling.

Caffeine can also have a detrimental effect on blood sugar. When caffeine is ingested, the nervous system is stimulated. Adrenaline is released and, in turn, the liver begins to emit stored blood sugar. Insulin is then released, and blood sugar drops below normal-a common seizure trigger for people with epilepsy.

The ultimate recommendation is to eliminate coffee or at the very least, limit the intake of coffee altogether.

Section 22:
Kitchen Essentials

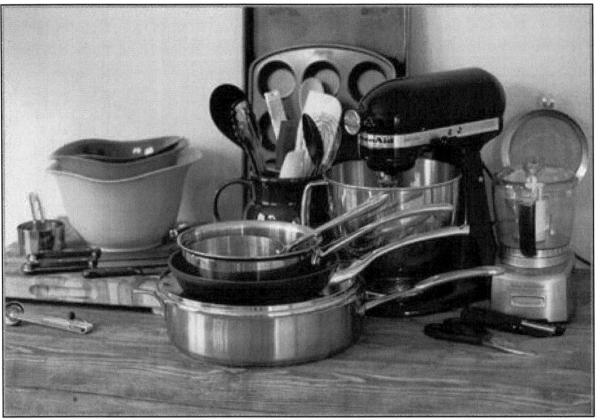

Now that you understand the truths about food, it's time to roll up your sleeves and get working. By now you might be thinking...."geez, do I have cook?" Many of you are intimidated by the prospect of cooking. Let me tell you, I was right there with you. I'm no gourmet cook, however, the more truths I got to know, the more I realized that my health is my own responsibility. I still have many family members and friends who look the other way if they think that I'm watching what they eat. They are secretly interested in what I have to say but scared to know that they might have to follow what I do. I give them little bits and pieces of information and boy do I get resistance. They get bent out of shape trying to defend the fact that they can't live in fear. The funny thing is that the next time I see them, they are doing one or more of the very thing we talked about last time, and they are a bit more informed about the truths about nutrition.

My husband and I have inside joke, "when in Rome, we must do what the Romans do." When we are visiting with friends and family, the last thing that we want to do is be picky about what we do or eat. We don't try to burden them with our criteria for good eating; we just give thanks and do things their way. Strangely, because they know me, they put the burden on themselves by trying hard to accommodate me. In order to be a good example, walk the talk and hold firm to your beliefs about what you are about to learn, however, change is hard for most people, including yourself, so be patient and just "go with the flow". You want them to be curious about what you are eating because you look so good and in good mood and energy, now because you are nagging. There is no right or wrong, it also does not make you better than them, just different in the way you approach and do things, it's your choice as it is their choice. Timing is everything when it comes to change. If you were trying to get me to do what I'm about to convince you to do, I would laugh in your face. I had a journey, my personal journey brought me here, just like your personal journey brought you to me. All is well...., no sense in judging.

The first thing my clients ask and the first thing I asked was, what do I need? In my experience, you can either succeed by design or fail by default. It takes a little intention to make this work.

Let's talk about the essentials:

Any kitchen will do for this program, from the tiny compact kitchen to a gourmet chef's kitchen. It's all about the intention of the cook who takes control. It's best to understand that the cook will be imparting its healing energy into the food when cooking. Therefore, first thing, let's get clean and keep it clean. Get rid of all clutter in the kitchen. Starting with the pantry, get rid of all the expired items, refined, and instant items that have a shelf life longer than you. All the sugared snacks and junk food that you've accumulated over the last few months or years, just toss it out. Clean out the refrigerator and get rid of all the unhealthy items that have been occupying the shelf, this stale food emanates negative energy that you don't need. Toss it out.

Create a space in the pantry for all the dry items. It's a good idea to organize the dried foods such as grains and beans in glass jars with good seals to maintain freshness. A good thing is to keep the ingredients easy to access to minimize the stress when you are cooking. For me, I keep the spices, oils, and condiments together, grains in one area, and the beans in their area. This allows me to clearly know where to find what I need when I need them as I cook.

Best part about cooking healthy is that we don't need fancy equipment or appliances. Below is the list of equipment that you may want to consider for your kitchen.

- Stainless Steel Cookware: Choose this over aluminum as the toxic metal can dissolve into the food with the aluminum. Recent research links Alzheimer's Disease and many other conditions.

- Stockpot: A large stockpot made of stainless steel or good quality enamel is a must.

- Cast-Iron Skillet: Heavy, old fashioned cast iron frying pans are great for all the sautéing and stir frying. Cast iron pans can be seasoned by not washing with soap but rinsed in hot water and dried in paper towels. Once seasoned in this manner, cast iron will never stick.

- Good Knives: This is essential for your kitchen. Keep your vegetable knives sharp at all times to keep your effort at ease when using your knife. I find that if the knife is dull, I don't enjoy cooking as much. Serrated knife for bread, steel knives for meats, and a large sharp knife for your vegetables is a good idea.

- Kitchen Scissors: A good quality kitchen scissor comes in very handy for variety of tasks such as snipping herbs and veggies to carving meats.

- Wooden Cutting Boards: Wooden cutting boards are less likely to harbor bacteria than the plastic ones. Two is recommended, one for meats and one for veggies.

- Handheld Blender and Mixer: This will come in handy in various tasks such as soup making right in the pot.

- Glass Food Container: Glass is my personal choice over stainless steel and plastic, you can easily see what's inside and don't have to worry about contamination.

- Wide Mouth Quart Size Mason Jars: This is great for storing jams, fermented products, and honey.

- Food Processor: This will make your slicing, grating, chopping, mixing and blending a breeze.

- <u>Stainless Steel Baking Pans and Cookie Sheets:</u> Again, better than the aluminum.

- <u>Mixer</u>: I like my vitamix mixer for various smoothies and for mixing various ingredients for soups for example. I find that this was well worth the money.

- <u>Juicer:</u> I have the Omega Juicer for fresh vegetable juice. I especially love this during the summer months.

Section 23:
Kitchen Tips

As you get in the habit of cooking, you'll find that these tidbits invaluable in keeping all things in line.

- Wash all fruits and vegetables in hydrogen peroxide or Clorox bleach (1 tsp per 1 Gallon), soak for 10 minutes and rinse.

- Avoid adding garlic to sautéing onions or other vegetables because it has a tendency to burn. Add garlic after you have added your liquid--stock, wine, stir-fry sauce, tomatoes, etc.

- Always use unsalted butter or make Ghee (See recipes)

- Use only celtic sea salt for your cooking.

- Use Extra Virgin Olive Oil, Grape seed Oil, Avocado Oil, and Ghee for cooking.

- Get in the habit of skimming foam off when making stock, beans, or stews. Add spices and seasoning after skimming the stock.

- Sauces and stews that contain wine should be boiled uncovered for 10 minutes to allow for the alcohol to evaporate.

- Grow your own herbs if you have garden space.

- Keep your kitchen uncluttered and your counters clear. Store only frequently used items in the kitchen cupboards and leave as much working space as possible on your counters.

- Use dishwasher powers with caution. Rinse twice as the residues are highly toxic.

- Get in the habit of planning ahead when preparing meals.

- Throw away all boxed cereals. Try soaked oatmeal or other grain, whole grain dishes such as pancakes, muffins, and fruit.

- Aim to use 50% vegetables, which are high in enzymes.

- Keep sweets to a minimum, even natural sweet.

Section 24:
Qi Metabolic Types

Four Qi Metabolic Types Defined:

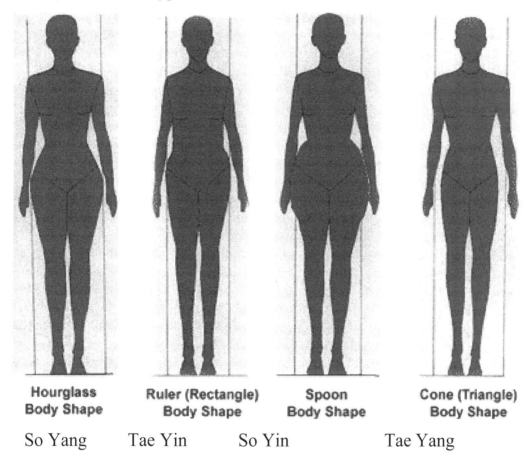

Hourglass Body Shape	Ruler (Rectangle) Body Shape	Spoon Body Shape	Cone (Triangle) Body Shape
So Yang	Tae Yin	So Yin	Tae Yang

The metabolic types have its foundation in "Sasang" Constitutional Medicine, which values the relationship between the mind and the body. The balance between Yin and Yang and the differences of "Qi," or life energy in internal organs depending on one of the S-Yang (hour glass type), S-Yin (Spoon Type), T-Yang (Cone Type) and T-Yin (Rectangle type) constitutions not only affects our physiological and metabolic status, but also results in differences in emotional characteristics, personalities and attitudes.

S-Yang (hour glass) Types:
Tend to be thin, with broad shoulders and narrow hips
S-Yang types are strong willed, and quick decision makers. They tend to be optimistic about everything, and do not hesitate to take on something new. If a new idea comes up, they tend to take immediate action. Such quick actions may mislead

others to thinking that things are rushed, but in the S-Yang type's mind, all plans are in place. S-Yang types are quick, multi-dimensional, and skilled at processing tasks.

However, S-Yang types tend to lack perseverance, and have difficulty finishing tasks that they started. Thus, an S-Yang type needs to have people around them who can hold them accountable. You can compare an S-Yang type to a sprint runner. They can spear forward with instantaneous speed, but cannot maintain their initial momentum over an extended period of time.

Recommended Foods :
Grains/Legumes: Barley, aduki beans, mung beans, kidney beans, buckwheat, green beans
Meat/Poultry: pork, duck, egg
Sea Foods: Oyster, sea cucumber, sea squirt, abalone, halibut, squid, octopus, crab, crayfish, swellfish, mackerel, mussel
Vegetables; Cabbage, cucumber, eggplant, squash, lettuce, burdock, carrot, celery, spinach
Fruits: Watermelon, melon, grapes, strawberries, bananas, pineapples, bananas, coconut, blueberries, persimmon, avocados

Foods To Avoid :
Hot foods and foods with high calories, Instant food or canned food, anything with artificial or chemical seasoning Chicken, beef, or milk, Wheat gluten, honey, goat, Peanuts, Red peppers, ginger, ginseng, green onions, mustard, spices like curry, wine, and coffee

T-Yang (Cone)Types:

T-Yang types are good communicators, and are sociable and decisive. Their positive and outward attitude allows them to communicate with and lead others. In comparison to other constitutions, T-Yang types are rather masculine in nature. They are decisive, and do not show regret once a decision is made. Since T-Yang types can be very charismatic, even to the extent of being self-righteous, they tend to possess leadership-qualities.

Recommended foods

Grains/legumes: buckwheat

Meat/Poultry: Avoid

Seafoods: fish, shrimp, oyster, ear shell, crab, octopus, cuttlefish (squid), sea cucumber, shellfish, mackerel, sea cucumber, sea squirt, prussian carp

Vegetables: celery, pine needles, Chinese cabbage, cucumber, lettuce

Proteins: Avoid poultry and meat;

Fruits: Grapes, persimmon, plum, cherries, kiwi

Avoid the following foods:

Spicy arid hot food, Fatty foods with high calories (sodas, ice cream, etc ...), ginger, onion, cinnamon, garlic, fennel, green onion, chives, turmeric, mustard, greasy foods, meats and poultry, honey, ginseng, hard liquor, and coffee

S-Yin (Spoon) Types:

SE types tend to be introverted, mild in temper and pay close attention to detail. They tend to have a strong sense of pride and are meticulous which can lead to a perfectionist character who does not like having mistakes. Generally, you can trust an S-Yin type person to be very independent. However, the pursuit of perfection can often mean that S-Yin types do not like doing two or more things at the same time, nor are they particularly good at completing tasks quickly. Their meticulous nature means that they want to deliberate carefully before reaching a conclusion. They can have tendencies of being indecisive. S-Yin typically does one task really well and does not do well with multi-tasking because then the care and time to do a perfect job is not possible.

S-Yin types are introverted; they do not outwardly express their anger or displeasure, and tend to suppress such feelings. Since anger needs to be vented, and suppressing it can lead to depression. Physiologically, their digestive functions are weaker in comparison, and with a slight increase in stress, S-YIn types can easily end up with indigestion and headaches.

Recommended Foods:

Grains/Legumes: rice, millet

Meat/Poultry/Diary: Chicken, lamb, goat, turkey, goat's milk

Sea Food: Pollack, swell fish, mudfish, snapper, yellow covina fish, anchovies, croaker fish, butterfish

Vegetables: Spinach, tomatoes, parsley, cabbage, green onions, garlic, ginger, red-peppers, mustard Black pepper, curry, sweet rice, millet, potatoes

Fruits: Jujubes, apples, oranges, and peaches, lemons, mangoes, nectarines, pomegranates, hawthorn berry

Tea: Ginger tea, ginseng tea, citron tea, cinnamon tea, honey tea

Foods to Avoid

Cold foods and high caloric foods, Buckwheat, cabbage, Beef, pork, milk, Pear, watermelon, melon, cucumber, raw fruits Sweet potatoes, chestnuts, walnuts

T-Yin (Rectangle):

T-Yin types are patient and poised. They tend to be persistent and see a task through to completion without difficulties. They can relax only when the task at hand is finished. Such patience and perseverance can lead to success in business.

T-Yin types tend to be introverted, and harbor ideas. They like to be sedentary and conservative.   Thus, they do not over-extend themselves, and takes on tasks that can be realistically completed. Their tendency to harbor things means that they are good at defending their own property and this desire can intensify and manifest itself as greed at times. T-Yin types have very realistic viewpoints, and can be calculating when it comes to considering their own benefits.

Recommended Foods:

Grains/Legumes: Wheat, brown rice, oats, soybeans, tofu, millet, lentils, beans, peas, peanuts

Meat/Poultry/Dairy: Beef, butter, cheese, yogurt, milk

Sea Food: Cod, eel, fish, salmon, tuna, cod fish

Vegetables: seaweed, kelp, marine plants, alfalfa sprouts, asparagus, bamboo shoots, bean sprouts, broccoli, carrots, cauliflower, mushrooms, pumpkin, radish, squash, sweet potatoes, taro, tomatoes, turnips, yams

Fruits/nuts: Pear, chestnut, walnut, ginkgo nuts, pine nuts, peanuts, plum, apricot

Foods to Avoid

High caloric foods, such as sodas, ice cream, and processed foods, Egg, chicken, Raw cabbage, apples Honey, sugar, ginseng, pork.

Section 25:
Qi Body Type Questionnaire

The following questionnaire aims to typify you into a category that is closest to your constitution. In Sasang Medicine, they look at the four key organs, lung, liver, spleen, and kidney, and the yang and yin balance to determine a person to enable the best health regimen for that individual. This dominance will determine the physiology of the individual and how they process the information received via sensory input and through food. This will give us insight to what information you need to balance your system, the more information we can gather, the greater ease and success we will be able to achieve.

The following questionnaire is designed to help you identify your body type. The questionnaire is divided up into four sections:

1st section: Will help determine your general mental and behavioral characteristics

2nd : Your personal business and social lives

3rd: your physical characteristics

4th: general health

Please read through the whole questionnaire and place a check next to each answer that best describes you. There are some overlaps and redundancies in the answers because some answers apply to more than one constitution. Please check all answers that apply to you. Try to relax, take your time, and really reflect on who you are and give an honest and unbiased answer. Determining the correct constitution will enable us to have you follow the program that is perfect for you and improve the outcome.

After you complete the questionnaire, count the number of checks in each column and total up the check marks. At the end of the questionnaire, there is a table for you to fill in your scores. Add up your scores from the four parts to find your overall totals, the highest number should be your constitution.

Ultimate Body Type Questionnaire

Part I: General Mental and Behavioral Characteristics

Tae-Yang	So-Yang	Tae-Yin	So-Yin
Resolute	Cheerful	Magnanimous	Crafty
Dogmatic	Mischievous	Prudent	Indecisive
Arrogant	Decisive	Taciturn	Introverted
Self righteous	Extroverted	Stubborn	Timid
Creative	Quick to Act	Ambitious	Decorous
Ingenuous	Brave	Decorous	Stubborn
Revolutionary	Righteous	Persistent	Meticulous
Charismatic	Risk taker	Tenacious	Deeply Reflective
Strong		Proper	Meditative
Leadership			

Appearance/General Impression

Fearless	Sharp	Benevolent	Soft
Arrogant	Intelligent	Dignified	Gentle
Neat	Riotous	Reserved	Calm
Elegant			Detail oriented
			Tidy

Which of the characteristics describes You at your best?

Benevolent	Life of the Party	Magnanimous	Precise
Compassionate	Quick Reasoning	Prudent	Methodical
Strong Leader	Quick Decision	Taciturn	Frank/Candid
Pioneering	Outspoken	Stubborn	Prudent
Original	Altruistic	Ambitious	Considerate
Courageous	Optimistic	Decorous	Non-contentious
Optimistic	Passionate	Persistent	Patient
Reformer	Worker	Tenacious	Persevering

Which of the characteristics describes You at worst

Dictator	Fickle	Greedy	Selfish
Rebellious	Rash/Impulsive	Selfish	Pessimistic
Uncooperative	Impatient	Lazy	Jealous/envious
Easily Angered	Persistent	Wicked	Procrastinating
Rude/Impertinent	Angry	Cowardly	Moody/Silent
Debauching	Belligerent	Overly Cautious	Nervous/
Urgent	Vain	Closed Minded	Apprehensive
Antisocial	Show of	Pleasure Seeking	Stingy
Outcast	Prodigal	Procrastinating	
	Neglectful of		
	family Domestic		

Total (   )   Total (   )   Total (   )   Total (   )

Part II: Personal, Business, and Social Life

| Tae-Yang | So-Yang | Tae-Yin | So-Yin |

1. How do you handle your personal and business work?

Tae-Yang	So-Yang	Tae-Yin	So-Yin
I am always resolute and firm in starting and finishing projects, no matter what.	I am quick in starting new projects, but seldom finish anything	I am a slow starter, but once the ball gets rolling, I carry things through to the end	I wait until I am certain of success before starting anything, but I usually finish what I start
I do things on a grand scale quickly, and without planning	I like to get things done quickly because I get bored easily	Slow, steady, and easy-does it is my approach to work	I am precise and meticulous in my work
I cannot sit still or work on one thing for an extended period of time	I cannot sit still or work on one thing for an extended period of time.	I can sit and work patiently in one location for a long time.	I can sit and work patiently in one location for a long time.

2. Your response to a new situation is:

Ready or not, here I come! I create new situations.	I am optimistic and enthusiastic in new and unfamiliar situations	Though I don't enjoy them, I am steady and reliable in unfamiliar situations	I am self protective in any situation, especially new and unfamiliar ones.

3. How do you respond in opportunity?

I make my own opportunities	When I see an opportunity, I quickly go after it .	I wait patiently for opportunities to arise. When they are within my reach, I grasp them tightly, and never let go	I wait and wait and lose my chance .

4. How do you generally make decisions?

I resolutely make my decisions and they are always correct	I quickly make decisions without weighing the pros and cons	I ponder over all decisions slowly, cautiously, and thoroughly	I am indecisive by nature, and prefer to defer decision making to others

5. Appearing or speaking before a crowd or relating to strangers;

| I make my presence known to everyone (even strangers) in the same manner

I say whatever comes to mind whenever I want to

I enjoy being the center of attention | I feel comfortable appearing or speaking before an audience

I say whatever comes to mind whenever I want to

I enjoy attention, and actively seek it. | I experience difficulty appearing or speaking before an audience

I do not speak until I feel certain that my ideas are correct

I don't try to stand out (but I wish people notice me) | I experience difficulty appearing or speaking before an audience

I do not speak until I feel certain that my ideas are correct

I shy away from the attention of others |

6. How do I generally respond to stress?

| Anger/Rage
Aggression
Stoically "take it"
Take Action | Irritability
Anger
Anxiety
Take Action | Fear
Procrastination
Lethargy
Conservatism | Procrastination
Insecurity
Anxiety/Worry
Indecisiveness |

7. Your personal and social relationships:

I can meet and talk to anyone, anytime Although I know many people, I really do not have any close friends. My friends must share my ideals	I enjoy going out and meeting new people; I love parties and crowds I'm not picky about making new friends, and do so with ease and enjoyment. Thus, I have many friends	I like meeting new people, but I'd rather spend time with family and friends I can easily make friends with anyone, and have good relationships with everyone	I have difficulty meeting new people, whether for business or social reasons. I am picky in forming friendships, and socialize only with those with whom I share a close affinity

8. On making mistakes

I never make mistakes. Mistakes are due to others, and I criticize them for it. (Even if I do make a mistake, I never regret it)	I often make mistakes, but I quickly forget about it. I can easily forgive others when they make mistakes	I work slowly, and rarely make mistakes. When there is a mistake, I can easily forgive myself or others for it.	I hate making mistakes, so I approach work carefully. I have a hard time forgiving mistakes in either myself or others.

9. When I fail

It is never my fault. It is always someone else's fault	I quickly forget about it and plan my next move	I get down on myself but come back no matter what it takes	I worry and stay depressed for a long time. It's hard for me to start fresh again

10. When someone mistreats you

I explode on the spot, no matter who the person is	I let my anger show, and shout and retort right back at the person	I dismiss it or talk things out. Although I may be hurt, I pretend I'm fine.	I get angry and annoyed, but I usually just back away.

Total (   )   Total (   )   Total (   )   Total (   )

Part III: Physical Characteristics

	Tae-Yang	So-Yang	Tae-Yin	So-Yin
Overall Body Structure	Thin body with large head Body resembles inverted triangle with narrow waist	Average sized body with medium sized bones Body resembles inverted triangle with wide, athletic shoulders and narrow hips/buttocks	Large sized body with thick bones and stocky build Greater waist and lower body development; either obese with pot-belly, or overall strong and heavy appearance	Small sized body with thin bones Body resembles ladder; well-developed hips, buttocks, and lower body with narrow shoulders and chest; but overall well balanced
Head size and shape	Large head, bulging at the crown/thick stiff neck	Protruding forehead and back of head	Large and round or large and square head	round or thin oval head

	Tae-Yang	So-Yang	Tae-Yin	So-Yin
Overall Facial Feature	Strong, intimidating look; or elegant, neat appearance

Wide forehead and protruding cheeks | Sensitive, but bright and animated

Small thin lips; sharp chin | Serene and dignified

Fleshy, large face; round, large nose; thick lips | Gentle and quiet or nervous and timid

Overall face small; small features, but well-balanced |
Eyes	Crystal-like, fierce, piercing, intimidating	Clear and sparkling or sharp and intense	Large, cow like, or large and bright	Pleasant, gentle, without focus (sleepy eyes)
Skin	Soft	Solid and thick; fairly rough; large skin pores	Solid, and thick; fairly rough; large skin pores	Soft and tender; slightly moist and swollen; small skin pores
Voice	Harsh, metallic; or sonorous overflowing with vigor	Clear and crisp	Thick, impure (muffled) and heavy	Somewhat calm, quiet and gentle

	Tae-Yang	So-Yang	Tae-Yin	So-Yin
Walk/Gait	Light and weak; straight stiff posture, resembling a robot	Straight posture; light and fast tempo; whole body shakes (looks unstable)	Slow and stable with measured gait (heavy regal steps)	Natural and gentle; careful and stable; may walk with upper body leaning forward
Part III	Total ( )	Total ( )	Total ( )	Total ( )

Park IV: General and Health Questions

Tae-Yang   So-Yang   Tae-Yin   So Yin

1. How is your general bowel movement?

I usually pass a great amount of large, well formed stool I can sometimes be constipated up to 6 or 7 days without problems, but if it goes over a week, then it bothers me.	I tend to get constipated easily I have a hard time dealing with constipation; it can make my chest feel hot and congested	I tend to get constipated and it makes me feel somewhat uncomfortable I tend to have alternating diarrhea and constipation, but it doesn't bother me.	I tend to get diarrhea easily and it really makes me tired I am usually constipated for 3 days, but it doesn't bother me.

2. How much do you generally sweat and how do you feel better after sweating profusely?

I don't sweat much and I feel okay after sweating	I don't sweat much and I feel okay after sweating	I tend to sweat a lot and feel energized when I do. I love sitting in saunas for long periods of time	I generally do not sweat much and feel very tired when I do. I do not generally like sitting in saunas.

164

3. What type of foods and drinks do you like?

Vegetables and fruits, raw and undercooked foods	All types of foods, but especially cool and cold foods (salads, vegetables, fruits)	Everything	Hot, spicy, warm, and well-cooked foods
Cool or cold drinks	Cold drinks or cool foods	Room temperature or cold drinks	Room temperature or warm drinks

4. What seasons do you like?

Cool, Cold Seasons	Cool/ Cold seasons	Any season except hot and damp	Warm/ hot season

5. Your manner of speech

Urgent	Fast, Garrulous	Usually Taciturn, but once I start, I talk in a cheerful manner	Usually quiet, but I talk a lot with people who are close

6. From which of the following ailments or conditions do you frequently suffer?

Vomiting	Urination or sexual problems	Palpitations	Indigestion
Weakness in waist and legs	Forgetfulness	Weak lungs	Sighing
	Constipation	Hypertension	Low energy
			Abdominal Pain
Difficulty swallowing	Low back pain	Weight Gain	
Hiccups			

Total (   )   Total (   )   Total (   )   Total (   )

Now total up the scores from Tae Yang, So Yang, Tae Yin, So Yin and the highest number in any category is your dominant constitution. Please note the questions were in the order of constitution as written above.

Tae Yang (   )

So Yang (   )

Tae Yin   (   )

So Yin   (   )

Section 26:
Why Eat Organic?

Why Eat Organic Foods?

Adopting an organic lifestyle helps to enhance the health of ecosystems and organisms. It is generally agreed upon by its supporters that growing and eating organic food is better for the environment. Growing foods organically excludes, when possible, the use of synthetic fertilizers, pesticides, growth regulators, and additives to livestock feed. Organic farmers usually rely on crop rotation and animal manures to maintain soil productivity, to supply plant nutrients, and to control weeds, insects, and other pests.

As a result, in addition to reducing your exposure to harmful pesticides, eating organically may also reduce your exposure to hormones, antibiotics, and potentially harmful irradiated food. Less antibiotic use may help to avoid the development of antibiotic resistance. according to the Environmental Working Group, (a non-profit organization that focuses on protecting public health and the environment regarding public policy), scientists have begun to agree that even small doses of pesticides and other chemicals can have long-term health consequences that begin during fetal development and early childhood.

The Organic Seal of Approval guarantees the consumer that there has been no usage of genetically modified crops or sewage sludge as fertilizer, helping to reduce toxic runoff into rivers and lakes and the subsequent contamination of watersheds and drinking water.

When you eat organically grown food, you may also be supporting small, local farmers, who are able to use less energy in transporting food from the field to the table.

Organic beef, chicken, and poultry are raised on 100% organic feed and never given antibiotics or hormones; in addition, their meat is never irradiated. Organic milk and eggs come from animals not given antibiotics or hormones and fed 100% organic feed for the previous 12 months. (Free-range eggs come from hens that are allowed to roam, but they are not guaranteed to be organic.)

Several studies support the claim that organic diets can dramatically reduce pesticide exposure. One such study compared pesticide metabolite levels in 18 children who got at least 75% of their juice and produce servings from organic sources with those in 21 children who got at least 75% of their juice and produce from conventionally grown food. Levels of organophosphorus pesticide metabolites in the urine collected were six to nine times higher in the children who ate conventionally grown foods than in those who ate organic diets.[1] More recent studies have corroborated these claims.[2-4]

Claims of enhanced nutritional benefits of organic foods have caused much controversy. However, studies have been able to support this claim. The Journal of Alternative and Complementary Medicine reported one study showing that, on average, organic crops contain 86% more chromium, 29% more magnesium, 27% more vitamin C, 21% more iron, 26% more calcium, 42% more manganese, 498% more iodine, and 372% more selenium. Significantly less nitrates were also found in the organic foods.[5] Resulting from nitrogen-based fertilizers, high nitrates in food and drinking water can be converted to potentially carcinogenic nitrosamines.

The Journal of Agriculture and Food Chemistry reported that organically grown corn, strawberries, and marionberries have significantly higher levels of anticancer antioxidants than nonorganically grown foods. Protective compounds, such as flavonoids, are produced by plants to act as their natural defense in response to stresses, such as insects or other competitive plants. The report suggested that good soil nutrition seems to increase the amount of these protective compounds, while pesticides and herbicides disturb their production.[6] A more recent study found similar results.[2]

Another important issue was brought to light in a 2010 review of studies that found an increased incidence of thyroid disease and diabetes with exposure to organochlorines.[7] The Environmental Working Group continues to stay on top of these issues as they come to the forefront.

What foods are most important to eat organically? Organic meats and dairy are appear to be the most heavily contaminated with hormones, pesticides and herbicides. Produce can be quite variable. If you are unable to eat organic produce, it is wise to be aware of those products that are the least contaminated with pesticides.

The Environmental Working Group publishes the lists below (Dirty Dozen™ and Clean 15 ™); they are updated annually. Foods are listed in order of importance. Their lists may be downloaded on ewg.org.

Genetically-modified Produce:

In order to determine if produce has been genetically modified, check the number PLU (product look-up) code on the sticker on most produce. If the number code is simply four digits, the produce is conventionally grown, which means it is not genetically modified and not organic. If the PLU code is a five digit code beginning with an "8", the product has been genetically modified. If the PLU code is a five digit code beginning with a "9", the product is organic, and also, by definition of organic, not genetically modified.

Section 27:
Food Journal Template

Day 1 Measurements

Measurements	Day 1	Day 10	Note
Chest			At nipple height
Waist			At the belly button
Hips			Largest Area of hips
Thighs			Largest circumference thigh
Body Weight			

DATE STARTED (date started program): _____

DATE FINISHED (date completed program_____

Exercise/Food Diary

Yes, its necessary because you are going to find that merely keeping track of all things going into your mouth makes you much more "aware" of your patterned behavior. We can only change our behavior if we know what our auto pilot behaviors are. You'll find some interesting patterns in what you are eating vs. what is going on in your day, specifically how you are feeling as a result of those events. My experience as a registered dietitian overseeing the various diet program reveals that this information is not accurate, however, clients get tremendous benefit from keeping a diary simply due to accountability. Just consider this a way to get to know you. Keep in mind that this 10 day challenge is a short challenge, however, it is my goal to have you change your behavior for the long term. The above numbers might not be a drastic as you'd hoped, however, I assure you that the way your cloths fit you might tell a different story.

It is a known fact that only 1/10 of our mental capacity is our "conscious" and 9/10 of it is "subconscious". We need to master our "subconscious" mind in order for any diet or exercise plan to be effective. Every detail of this program has taken this into consideration, the self-affirmations are very important part of this challenge. Our physical body is the manifestations of our thoughts, that is why I wanted you to visualize yourself in your favorite outfit in the weight that you desire, if the mind can conceive, it can achieve. I need to align you with your mental image of yourself with your goal, otherwise, you are setting yourself up for failure.

Research also proves that the diet program or any other self-improvement programs cannot be successful by will power alone because our will power is the "conscious" mind, which is only the 1/10 of your mind. It is the "subconscious mind" that we must tap into to have lasting changes. I assure you that once you tap into it, the process of losing weight or changing any behavior will be a piece of cake.

Through this program I want you to align yourself with the "special" you that you may not know exists inside of you. I want the ultimate success for you in all areas of your life, both wealth, health, and relationships. You have invested in so much more than a mere diet, but a very personalized clinical approach from an experienced clinician who's been through the mind body control. As a healer, I believe I need to approach every patient as a whole person, mind, body, and spirit, otherwise I set myself up for limited benefit or ultimate failure to impact my patients.

Please follow through with keeping the diary and do not deviate from the specific program I've put together for you.

I've also included your emotional feelings into the diary so that you may realize your patterned thoughts. Once you know, you can change your thoughts. You are what you eat and what you think.

Date _____

Three things you are grateful for: (ie. Thank you for the fresh air, for my family, for the sun that is shining brightly, for the food, water, car, work........., anything goes.

1._____

_____

2._____

_____

3._____

_____

Positive Affirmations: (ie. I can be all that I can be. I feel and look my very best. I am a special being here on earth for a grand purpose., etc.)

1._____

_____

2._____

_____

3._____

_____

Time	Meal/Specific Food Eaten	Portion	Feelings (Do I feel stressed, happy, tired, confused, guilty, etc.)
	Breakfast: _____ _____ _____ _____ _____ _____ _____ _____ _____ _____ _____ _____		
	Snack: _____ _____ _____ _____	_____ _____ _____ _____ _____ _____	_____ _____ _____ _____ _____ _____

Time	Meal/Specific Food Eaten	Portion	Feelings (Do I feel stressed, happy, tired, confused, guilty, etc.)
	Lunch: _____ _____ _____ _____ _____ _____ _____ _____ _____ _____ _____ _____ _____	_____ _____ _____ _____ _____ _____	_____ _____ _____ _____ _____ _____ _____ _____ _____ _____ _____ _____ _____ _____
	Snack: _____ _____ _____ _____ _____		_____ _____ _____ _____ _____ _____ _____ _____

Time	Meal/Specific Food Eaten	Portion	Feelings (Do I feel stressed, happy, tired, confused, guilty, etc.)
	Dinner:		
	Snack:		

Water Intake: Goal _____

Actual _____

Exercises

Exercise	Frequency	Cardio/Walk/Eliptical, Treadmill/Bike

Comments/Notes:

Today's observation of my behavior:

What are my triggers? (things or events that trigger me to eat out of emotion, not due to hunger and nourishment)

My best accomplishments:

Section 28:
Alkaline Energy Guide

<u>Ultimate Energy Guide</u>

So many of my patients and clients complain of low energy level and uncontrollable weight gain. In fact I feel that low energy is the root of all evil because if you are tired, then you can forget about cooking, preparing, let alone exercising. It puts us in a frame of mind that is set up for failure. That is why I wanted to share ways to give you the ultimate boost in energy to help you conquer all that life has to throw at you. Our body is our temple, it's something to be taken care of to optimize its performance. I've tabulated a 8 step energy guide below to shed some light on simple things that you can do today to improve your energy and as a side effect, lose weight!

1. <u>Eliminate all High-sugar foods</u>:   There is evidence that refined sugar contributes to obesity, nutrient deficiencies, and hypoglycemia. It also appears to play a role in increasing cholesterol levels, decreasing HDL (good cholesterol), and the development of diabetes.

There are some sweetener choices that are better than others. Generally an added sweetener that has a "low glycemic index" (GI) – one that does not elicit a spike in blood sugar – is preferable.

Brown rice syrup. It is thought that the glucose from this sweetener is released into the blood stream more slowly than from white sugar for example.

Honey is a more natural sweetener, is less processed than most, with many health benefits, but its GI is not low.

agave nectar, proven to have a very low GI. However, there have been claims that agave is no better than high fructose corn syrup. This may not be true if you use the organic form of agave.

While molasses is more refined, blackstrap molasses does have a significant amount of iron, calcium, potassium, and B vitamins.

Fruit concentrates, such as apple juice concentrate, contain more nutrients than refined sugar, but lend a sweet flavor.

Stevia is a powdered herbal sweetener that has no effect on blood sugar and is many times sweeter than white sugar.

Sugar content in any given processed food can be confusing. Read the labels, sugar is any of the following; High fructose corn syrup (HFCS), glucose, fructose, maple syrup, brown rice syrup, barley malt, dextrose, molasses, sorbitol, evaporated cane juice, sucralose, honey, brown sugar. A product may contain more than one kind of sugar. When making choices, choose lower glycemic index and/or naturally occurring sweets over refined sweets, e.g., fruit juice/fruit, pure maple syrup, brown rice syrup, barley malt, stevia, or agave nectar.

Stay away from artificial sweeteners that can cause inflammation and zap the energy out of you such as aspartame (Nutra Sweet) or sucralose (Splenda).

Hints to keep added sugars to a minimum: Ingredients are listed by weight in descending order. Sweeteners should never be one of the first ingredients. Avoid a food if sugars are not listed toward the end in the list of ingredients (if at all).

2. Limit intake of High-fat foods: Especially foods with arachidonic acid and saturated fats (dairy and animal fat primarily)

a. For medium-heat cooking, use olive oil or short or medium chain natural saturated fats, like coconut oil. These oils are more stable and don't have the health risks associated with hydrogenated processed saturated fats. It is best to keep high heat or deep frying to a minimum since EFAs are destroyed with cooking. When you do cook with oils over higher heat, it is best to use a high oleic safflower oil as this is most stable under higher heat conditions. Add healthy monounsaturated and polyunsaturated fats to your foods. The best to use is cold-pressed extra-virgin olive oil, along with sesame (tahini), flax, walnut, almond, grapeseed, and avocado oils.

b. Avoid ALL processed fats. This means margarine, processed baked goods and chips – anything labeled "hydrogenated" or "partially hydrogenated." These are unnatural damaged fats and there is absolutely nothing good about them. If you have to choose between butter and margarine, choose butter especially ghee, (and use it sparingly). Smart Balance and Earth Balance are two newer margarines that contain healthier oils with no trans-fats.

c. Keep consumption of animal-derived saturated fat to a minimum. Avoid fatty cuts of meat, items cooked or prepared with high amounts of saturated fats. Small amounts of the short or medium chain saturated fats, such as coconut oil are acceptable.

d. Purchase good quality oils. It is important that they be labeled "cold-pressed" so they are not exposed to high heat and chemical alteration. These oils should be kept in tinted, glass bottles with a tight lid, refrigerated and not used for high heat frying. Additionally, olive oil should be labeled "extra-virgin" or "first-pressing." Coconut oil should be labeled both "organic" and "virgin."

3. <u>Food Allergens</u>: Check to make sure that you don't have any food allergies or sensitivities because theses can form immune complexes and lead to inflammation and cause you to become fatigue. Try eliminating the common allergic foods like peanuts, gluten, soy, refined foods, red meat, caffeine, and alcohol.

4. <u>Insufficiency of fiber</u>: Eat plenty of fruits, vegetables, nuts and seeds because they contain ample amounts of phytonutrients, antioxidants, vitamins, and minerals that are readily absorbed by our gut. Eating foods high in fiber in this ways pulls toxins from the GI tract and acts like a broom to sweep them out keeping a nice clean intestinal surface to keep the barrier to both protect and nourish our body.

5. <u>Exercise at least 3 X week</u>: 1) Exercise helps to decrease adipose tissue (fat) which can zap the energy out of us and 2) Exercising muscle reduces inflammation improves insulin sensitivity leaving us ever so energized. 3. Exercise also increase endorphin release which give us mental clarity and improve energy.

6. <u>Ensure Vitamin D levels are adequate</u>:

a.   Vitamin D is probably the most underutilized treatment in modern medicine!

b. There are two ways to get Vitamin D- to eat it in the diet, or to make it in the skin. The skin reaction will not occur without exposure to UV-B light- which is blocked by sunscreen use.

c. Vitamin D is made from cholesterol, like other sex steroid hormones. Chemically, it very closely resembles estrogen and testosterone, and it is probably better called a pro-hormone than a vitamin!

d. Symptoms of Vitamin D deficiency can be very subtle: fatigue, muscle cramps or weakness, poor balance, inability to get up from a chair without pushing on the armrests, fragile nails, depression and bone fracture.

VITAMIN D REPLACEMENT

e. Before embarking on Vitamin D replacement, you must know your Vitamin D level.

The best test is a 25-(OH) Vitamin D level. Optimal levels are 50-60 ng/ml. 32-50 is low normal. 20-32 is deficient, and <20 is severely deficient. A 1,25-(OH) Vitamin D test is also available, but does not correlate to most disease states because of its short half-life.

Vitamin D supplementation should never be undertaken without a target in mind, and with the knowledge that calcium and magnesium intake is sufficient and/or supplemented at the same time.

Make sure to seek medical advice to know your needs with Vitamin D.

7. Ensure Vitamin and Mineral supplementation: Due to the less than ideal soil today in the industrialized populations, our foods contain less nutrients than in the past. Especially magnesium, deficiency of which is seen in 20-40% of most "industrialized" populations. It's a good idea to supplement your diet with a good quality, pure multivitamin with B-complexes, zinc, and magnesium.

8. Learn to cope with Emotional stress: Exercise, meditate, journal, and take Epson baths as recommended in my program to manage the stresses in your life. Our world today is very chaotic and stressful. We need to be aware of our thoughts and behaviors to make sure that we provide ourselves with an outlet to deal and cope. Stress can Promote inflammation, impair wound healing, and promote immunosupbresion which can ultimately sap you of energy.

Number one complaint in my clinical practice is how tired my patients are. I find that small steps can have profound effects in people's behavior and attitudes. You will find that if you follow my plan, you will have so much vitality, energy, and zest for life like never before. Good luck.

Section 29:
Anti-Inflammatory Diet Guide

Growing body of evidence suggest that low grade inflammation over time can ultimately lead to disease. In fact, all diseased states are as a result of inflammation. We know that inflammation is the redness, swelling, and the heat that the body produces but at a deeper level, sometimes the inflammation can be felt as a muscle, bone, or joint pain, fatigue, or breathing difficulties just to give some perspective.

I have Lupus, which is a auto-immune disrupted disease that causes secondary inflammation that not only ages me quicker, but the pain that I have really makes it difficult to keep moving. I have an interest in this area because I feel that if I can keep my inflammation down by feeding my body nourishment that are anti-inflammatory then I won't need to resort to medications to keep the pain at bay.

Below is a detailed guide along with the recipes to help you to eat healthy by eating foods that are anti-inflammatory.

BREAKFASTS

1-2 omega 3 rich eggs, scrambled with olive oil (1 tsp or olive oil spray) and onions and peppers and cilantro garnish. One apple or pear with herbal or decaf tea

½ to 1 cup old fashioned or steel-cut oats. Mix in 2 Tb walnuts, 1t.flaxseed oil or1- 2 T. ground flax seed, 1/2 cup berries. almond or rice milk to taste

1 cup plain organic yogurt with 2-3 Tbs. walnuts or pecans, 1t stevia (if desired), 1 tsp. Cinnamon, 1/2 cup berries or 1 small apple, cut into chunks. Cover fruit in 1T lemon juice before adding to yogurt if desired.

Berry smoothies* (see recipes)

LUNCHES

4oz chicken breast, sautéed with 1 tsp or spray olive oil (salt and pepper, fresh-squeezed lime juice and cilantro. One cup cooked black beans, topped with guacamole* (see recipe).

Large salad with 2-3 cups spring mix. Add red onion slices, 2 Tbs. pumpkin or sunflower seeds, cucumber, broccoli and top with 2-3 oz lean meat or 1 hardboiled egg and ½ cup beans. Add 2T healthy oil based salad dressing *(see recipe) and a side of fruit - apple, orange or pear.

Bowl of chicken and rice soup with vegetables. Add a side salad with 1-2 cups of greens, 1-2T olive oil and balsamic vinegar dressing and an apple or orange on the side.

4-6oz. sautéed chicken breast with side of slaw made with cabbage and/or broccoli slaw, zesty Italian dressing and toasted slivered almonds. Add an orange or apple to the side.

1-2 cups Vegetable soup*(see recipe-easy to make ahead on a weekend and eat on all week), whole grain rice cake, 1 Tbs. almond butter sprinkled with 1 Tbs. sunflower seed nuts and/or ½ cup blueberries on top.

DINNERS

4-6oz sirloin, cooked to preference, ½ to 1 cup brown rice with side of roasted Brussels sprouts* (see recipe)

4-6oz salmon filet, sautéed or broiled with 1 tsp. olive oil per fillet, lemon slice and salt and pepper to taste. Sautéed broccoli with garlic and ½ to1 cup wild rice (if desired) to the side.

4-6oz Lamb chop, 1 baked sweet potato, side of spinach and garlic salad* (see recipe)

Chicken or beef fried rice - Cook brown rice and once done, add to cooked cut up chicken or beef then sauté one egg into the rice with some 2-3 tsp sesame oil. Add broccoli and other vegetables to taste.

SNACKS

¼ cup nuts plus 2T dried fruit

1 apple with 1-2T almond butter

Rice cakes with 1-2 T. almond or cashew butter

Hummus or guacamole and vegetables, corn chips or crackers *(see recipes)

Homemade pickles - cucumber and onion slices with 1 tsp. Sea salt and 1-2 tsp. Fresh or dry dill, 1/2 apple cider vinegar and 1/2 water mixture

Cinnamon apples - cut up an apple and add cinnamon and stevia and microwave for 45 seconds

Balsamic vinegar and fruit *(see recipe)

DRINKS

Filtered water, sparkling mineral water, seltzer water and misc. teas esp. green tea and herbal tea

OTHER LUNCH and DINNER OPTIONS:

Vegetarian Spaghetti Squash* (see recipe- may use 2 large -29 oz. canned petite diced tomatoes for the 10 fresh roma tomatoes if desired. Low sodium or no salt added if possible)

Portobello Steaks * (see recipe) serve with roasted or grilled veggies or a baked sweet potato.

RECIPES

BREAKFAST

Nut Butter Oatmeal: Place 1 cup water, 1/3 cup steel cut or old fashioned oats and 2-3 chopped dates or 2T raisins in small saucepan. Bring to a boil. Reduce heat and simmer, stirring occasionally, for about 5 minutes. Add 1-2T peanut or almond butter and mix well. Serve with 1 grated apple and a dollop of plain yogurt if desired.

Apple Oatmeal: Place 1 cup steel cut or old fashioned rolled oats, 2 cups water, 2 small apples, washed and cut into bite sized pieces, 1/4 cup raisins or no sugar added dried berries and 1 tsp cinnamon if desired together in a saucepan. Cover and cook over low heat for 20 minutes stirring occasionally. (This makes 2-3 servings)

Homemade Granola: Mix together the following: 1 pound rolled oats, 2 cups oat bran, 1 cup grated coconut, 1 cup chopped pecans, 1/4 cup sesame seeds, 1/2 cup sunflower seeds, 1/3 cup oil, 1/2 cup agave nectar or stevia to taste. Spread a thin layer about 1/2" thick on an un-oiled cookie sheet and bake at 350 degrees F for 20 min or until golden brown. Stir occasionally during the baking to assure even browning. Remove from oven and add non sweetened dried fruit if desired; mix well. Let cool before storing. (This makes many servings and limit to ½ cup portion per meal. Serve dry or with almond or rice milk.)

Berry Smoothie: Blend in a blender: 1 cup rice or almond milk, 1-2 scoop powdered protein of choice to equal approx. 15-25 grams protein,1/2 cup ice cubes if not using frozen fruit, 1/2 cup strawberries, 1/2 cup blueberries, 1-2 T gd. Flax seed, 1 -2 T (optional) nut butter.

Super Smoothie: 1 cup Cran Water (Diluted 100% natural cranberry Juice), ¼ cup fresh or frozen cranberries, ¾ cup frozen blue berries, 1 scoop whey protein, 1 Tbs. flax oil, 1 Tbs. ground flax seed, stevia to taste if desired. Combine all ingredients in the blender. Mix until smooth and creamy or about 1-2 minutes. (Change to strawberries and raspberries instead of blueberries for variety and/or add ½- cup plain yogurt instead of whey protein if desired)

Oat Crepes: Place 1/3 cup rolled oats, 1/3 cup almond or rice milk and 1 egg in the blender and blend until smooth. The batter will be thin. Drop the batter by the 1/4 cup or less onto a hot lightly oiled skillet or crepe pan. Cook over medium-high heat until set and golden brown on the bottom. Turnover and cook briefly on the other side. Top with fresh berries and plain yogurt and 2 Tb. Pecans, walnuts or almonds if desired.

LUNCH and DINNER

Spinach and Garlic Salad: Place 1-2 garlic cloves into an ovenproof dish and add 2T olive oil. Roast in a 375 degree F oven for 15-20 min. Transfer the garlic and 2T olive oil into a salad bowl and add 1# organic spinach, 1/2 cup chopped walnuts, and 2 t lemon juice and toss well to coat the salad and season with salt and pepper to taste.

Stir-Fried Greens: Cut up 8 scallions, 2 celery stalks, 1 cup white radish and 1 1/2 cup sugar snap peas or snow peas into strips. Shred 1 1/2 cups Napa cabbage and 6oz. Bok Choy or spinach. Heat 1T olive oil and 1T sesame oil together in a wok and add the garlic. Add the other cut vegetables to the wok and stir-fry for about 2 minutes. Then add the cabbage and Bok Choy or spinach to the skillet and stir-fry for another minute or so. Add 1t finely grated fresh gingerroot and pepper to taste and cook another minute. This is great with kale and other misc. greens of your choosing.

Rice and Beans: Cook 1 cup brown or wild rice according the package directions and set aside. Heat 2T olive oil in a skillet and add green and red peppers one each, chopped, and one onion and cook for 5 minutes or until soft. Add 1 small red or green chili chopped and 2 chopped tomatoes and cook for another 2-3 minutes. Add this vegetable mixture and 1 cup canned red kidney beans, rinsed and drained, to the rice and blend. Add 1T chopped fresh basil and 2 t chopped fresh thyme and 1t Cajun spice (such as Tony Chachere's) and mix well. Sea salt and pepper to taste.

Black Bean Soup: In a 3 qt pot, heat 1T olive oil over medium heat, add 1 medium chopped onion and 2 minced garlic cloves and cook until tender. Stir in 2t chili powder, 1t ground cumin, 2 cans black beans, rinsed and drained, 1 can organic vegetable broth and 1 cups water and heat to boiling. Reduce heat to low and simmer for 15 minutes. Use a handheld mixer to blend the soup together to a creamy consistency. Garnish with 1/2 cup chopped cilantro and lime wedges. Add avocado for garnish as well, if desired.

Hot Lentil Salad: Cook one cup brown or green lentils according to package instructions. Heat 4T olive oil in a pan and cook one small sliced onion with 4 stalks of sliced celery, 2 garlic cloves, crushed or grated, 2 diced zucchini and 3/4 cup fresh green beans cut into small lengths. Cook for 5 minutes, then add 1/2 each of red bell pepper and yellow bell pepper, diced, into the pan and cook for another minute. Stir in 1t Dijon mustard and 1T balsamic vinegar. Pour the warm mixture over the cooked lentils and toss together well. Season with salt and pepper to taste.

Chicken Jambalaya: Cook 3 oz brown rice as directed on package and set aside. Heat 1-2T olive oil in a heavy skillet and cook two large (6-8oz) chicken breasts, diced, until brown, about 3 minutes on each side. Add another 1-2T olive oil to the pan and cook 2 cloves crushed garlic and 1 small red onion, chopped, for approx. 2-3 minutes. Add 1 diced eggplant, 1 diced green bell pepper, 1/2 cup frozen peas and 1 cup broccoli florets and cook for another 5 minutes. Stir in 1 cup organic vegetable broth, 8oz fresh or canned chopped tomatoes, 1T tomato paste, 1t Creole seasoning and 1/2t chili flakes. Add salt and pepper to taste and cook for 15-20 minutes. Stir in the rice and chicken and cook until hot.

Stuffed Peppers: Cut 4 green peppers in half and place in an oven-safe dish. Mix together 2 cups cooked long grain brown or wild rice, 1 can organic stewed tomatoes, one small onion, chopped, 1 cup chopped fresh mushrooms, 2T fresh basil and salt and pepper to taste. Stuff the pepper halves with the rice mixture so that each pepper contains an even amount of the rice mixture. Bake in the oven at 350 degrees for 30 minutes or until peppers are tender.

Vegetable Soup: In a large saucepan, sprayed with nonstick cooking spray, sauté 1 cup sliced carrots, 1 cup diced onion and 2-4 garlic cloves, minced, over low heat until soft, about 5 minutes. Add 4 cups (32 oz.) organic beef, chicken or vegetable broth, 2-3 cups diced green cabbage, 1 cup green beans, ½-1 can no salt added tomato paste, ½ t dried basil, ¼ t oregano and ¼ t salt; bring to a boil. Lower heat and simmer, covered, about 15 minutes or until beans are tender. Stir in ½ cup diced zucchini and heat 3-4 minutes. Serve hot. Add other vegetables, legumes etc. as desired.

Portobello Steaks:

6 Portobello mushroom caps

1/2 cup fresh squeezed lemon juice

2 tablespoons apple cider vinegar

2 tablespoons Pure Maple syrup

2 teaspoons fresh grated ginger

1/2 teaspoon marjoram

Wash mushrooms and place in a gallon size plastic sealable bag. Combine remaining ingredients in a bowl and stir to combine. Add to the mushrooms and marinate for a few hours. Grill indoors or out until cooked through.

Serve with baked sweet potatoes and grilled squash and asparagus.

Grilled Vegetables: Toss yellow squash, zucchini, and asparagus with 2 tablespoons extra-virgin olive oil. Salt and Pepper to taste. Grill indoors or out until tender.

Roasted Vegetables: Take a variety of raw non-starchy vegetables, washed and prepared in med sized portions. Fill 9 by 13 or roasting pan. Drizzle olive oil, minced garlic, small amt of sea salt, pepper to taste. Roast at 375-400 degrees for 20-30 min stirring every 15 min until desired tenderness. Enjoy!!

Baked Sweet Potatoes: Wash sweet potatoes, prick with a fork several times and place in a 400 degree oven for an hour. Less time may be needed if potatoes are small.

Vegetarian Spaghetti Squash: Slice squash in half lengthwise. Scoop out the seeds with a spoon as you would a pumpkin. Then completely submerge both halves in boiling water and cook for about 20 to 25 minutes, or until the inside is tender to a fork and pulls apart in strands. (It is better to undercook if you are not sure). Remove, drain, and cool with cold water or an ice bath to stop the cooking. Then use a fork to scrape the cooked squash out of its skin, and at the same time, fluff and separate the squash into spaghetti-like strands. Discard the skin. Reheat the squash strands by dipping with a strainer in boiling water just before serving.

You can also bake the spaghetti squash in the oven. Just scoop seeds out as described above and prick outside skin with a fork. Place skin side up in a baking pan with 1 inch water. Bake 45 minutes or until tender in a 400 degree oven. Remove and allow to cool for a few minutes until they can be handled. Scrape with a fork as mentioned above and serve with stir fried sauce.

Stir Fried Sauce

10 Roma tomatoes, peeled, seeded, and chopped coarsely(may use 2- 40 oz. Petite diced or crushed tomatoes, use no salt added if possible)

2 cups thinly sliced mushrooms

2 cloves garlic

2 cups chopped broccoli florets or 1 package baby spinach

2 teaspoons oregano (powdered or flakes)

Sea salt to taste

Sauté mushrooms and onion with garlic and oregano. Add tomatoes and other vegetables. Cook until tender and heated through. Toss in a large bowl with spaghetti squash strands. Serve hot. Approx. 6 servings.

SNACKS

Hummus: In a food processor, combine 2, 15oz cans garbanzo beans, drained and rinsed; 4 cloves mashed garlic, 2/3 cup tahini, 1/2 cup water, 1/4 cup olive oil and the juice of one large lemon. Blend until smooth. Add salt starting at 1/2t and add to taste. Place this hummus mixture into a serving dish and sprinkle with toasted pine nuts and chopped parsley. This can be served with carrots, celery, cucumbers, jicama, bell peppers or any other vegetables as well as blue corn chips or any type of healthy crackers. .

Guacamole: Cut two avocados in half and remove the pit. Scoop out flesh with a spoon and place in a food processor. Add 1/2 cup fresh cilantro, 1 clove garlic, juice of half a lemon and puree in the food processor. Add 4-5 chopped cherry tomatoes and season with sea salt to taste.

Homemade Pickles: Chop one large cucumber into slices and add half of a small sliced yellow onion and mix with 3-4T fresh dill. Place these ingredients in a mixture of one 1 cup apple cider vinegar and 1 cup water into a container with a tight lid. Let the cucumber and onion marinate for at least 4 hours in the refrigerator before eating. This will keep in the refrigerator for at least one week. Add sea salt and pepper to taste.

Cinnamon Apples: Cut up one medium red apple into cored slices and place in a microwave-safe dish. Add 1t cinnamon mixed with 1T water and pour over chopped apples and microwave for 45-60 seconds. Add one packet of stevia to the warmed apple if desired and enjoy.

Balsamic Vinegar and Fruit: Quarter 3-4 of your favorite stone fruits, such as peaches, plums or nectarines, removing the pit, and place in an oven-safe dish. Drizzle balsamic vinegar over the fruit and bake at 400 degrees for 15-20 minutes. Remove fruit and garnish with fresh mint leaves.

Roasted Nuts: Take 2 cups of your favorite nuts, preferably walnuts or pecans, and lightly coat with 1T olive oil. Spread nuts out onto a baking sheet and place in the oven for 10-12 min at 350 degrees. Stir nuts halfway through baking for even browning. Watch nuts carefully, they burn easily. Let nuts cool and add a small amount of sea salt to taste if desired. They are great even without salt.

Section 30:
The Dirty Dozen; Clean 15

2012 SHOPPER'S GUIDE TO PESTICIDES- THE DIRTY DOZEN & CLEAN 15

Source: Environmental Working Group (EWG)

Did you know that the fruits and vegetables at your grocery store could be covered with bug killers, fungicides and other chemicals?

In fact, the most recent round of U. S. Department of Agriculture and Food and Drug Administration tests have found detectible pesticide residues on 68 percent of food samples.

That's why EWG is committed to giving you the tools you need to buy safe and healthy produce for your family and have just updated their Shoppers Guide to Pesticides, Dirty Dozen and Clean 15 List.

The Shopper's Guide to Pesticides will help you to determine the which fruits and vegetables have the most pesticides residues and are the most important to buy organic. By avoiding the most contaminated fruits and vegetables and eating the least contaminated you can lower your pesticide intake substantially.

The Dirty Dozen (Buy these organic where possible):

1. Apples

2. Celery

3. Sweet bell peppers

4. Peaches

5. Strawberries

6. Nectarines – imported

7. Grapes

8. Spinach

9. Lettuce

10. Cucumbers

11. Blueberries – domestic

12. Potatoes

Plus: Green beans, Kale/Greens – May contain residues of special concern

The Clean 15 (Lowest is pesticides, ok to buy not organic when):

1. Onions

2. Sweet Corn

3. Pineapples

4. Avocado

5. Cabbage

6. Sweet Peas

7. Asparagus

8. Mangoes

9. Eggplant

10. Kiwi

11. Cantaloupe – domestic

12. Sweet Potatoes

13. Grapefruit

14. Watermelon

15. Mushrooms

Section 31:
Alkaline Recipes

<u>Whole Grains</u>

Whole Grains are considered the staple of whole foods diet. The grains sometimes get the bad reputation for being acidic in the spectrum of alkaline-acidity scale, however, the key thing is to combine the foods appropriately to ensure that every meal you bring balance. When prepared with the right combination, whole grains are very nourishing.

It can be very daunting to go to the whole foods store and find the various grains on the shelf. Don't be scared, just allow your creativity to awaken to the possibilities. Once purchased, grains should be stored in glass sealed jars in a cupboard or pantry. It may be a good idea to add a bay leaf to each jar to prevent grain moths. I recommend that you label each jar so that you know what they contain.

Whole Oat Porridge

9 oz whole oats

60 oz water

Handfuls of Raisons

1 Tbsp of honey

1 cup Berries

Handful of Walnuts (or nuts of your preference)

It is ideal to make it the night before. Wash the oats place in pot and add water. Bring oats to boil and boil for 30 minutes, Turn off the heat and leave the pot over night.

The oats will absorb water overnight, in the morning check to make sure that there is some water in the oats. If not, add some water to cover the oats. Stir and cook over low heat over low flame for 10-15 minutes. Switch off the heat and let rest. Spoon out one serving in a bowl, place fruits, nuts, and sweetener on top and garnish with mint if desired.

(Place the left over oats in a glass or stainless steel container and refrigerate them. Each morning, use for breakfast, add water and heat over low flame, you can vary the topping, i.e. nuts and fruits. You can also use seeds.)

Polenta Porridge with Yogurt

5 oz organic polenta

4 cups cold water

1 TBSP sunflower seeds

Yogurt to taste

Place polenta and water in saucepan. Cover and bring to a boil; uncover and reduce the heat to low and simmer for 10 minutes, stirring occasionally. Turn off the heat and place in a bowl, add yogurt and add sunflower seeds on top.

Squash and Short Grain Brown Rice

This is a nice dish in the fall and the winter. You can add some water and make this dish a porridge for breakfast, you will find that it'll supply you with a warming energy.

2 cups short grain brown rice, ideally rinsed and soaked at least an hour (drain, and discard the water)

1 cup cubed winter squash

3 cups filtered water

1 tsp sea salt

1 TBSP barley miso

1 Sheet toasted nori, slivered

1 TBSP parsley finely minced

Combine rice, squash and water and bring to a boil, lower heat to low and cook for 50 minutes.   Add the salt.

Puree miso in small amount of water and simmer it 3-4 minutes. When the rice is cooked, remove from heat and add the miso puree into the hot rice and transfer to a serving bowl. Garnish with nori and parsley and serve.

4-5 servings

Vegetable Fried Rice

1-2 tsp dark sesame oil

3-4 slices fresh ginger, cut into thin matchsticks

1-2 cloves fresh garlic, slivered

Sea salt

1/2 cup each onion, carrot, burdock, cut into matchsticks, thinly sliced button mushrooms and shredded cabbage

2 cups cooked short grain brown rice

1-2 stalks of broccoli, broken into florets, stems peeled and sliced

Soy sauce

Brown rice vinegar or organic apple cider vinegar

2-3 Sprigs flat-leaf parsley for garnish

Heat the oil in the skillet over medium low heat. Add the ginger, garlic, and a pinch of salt and stir until golden brown. Add the onions and add a pinch of salt and stir until the onion is translucent. Add the carrot, burdock and mushrooms and stir occasionally. Sir in the cabbage and cook until the cabbage begins to wilt.

Spread vegetables evenly over the skillet and top with cooked rice, then broccoli florets and stems. Add 1/4 cup of water to allow everything to steam together, cover and cook over medium heat until all water is absorbed, about 10 minutes. Turn off the heat and season to taste with rice vinegar. Stir and transfer to the serving bowl, garnish with parsley sprigs.

4 servings

Millet and Veggie Burgers

This dish is fun and perfect for snack or lunch.

1-2 tsp avocado oil

3-4 slices of ginger , cut into thin matchsticks

Sea salt

1 cup millet, rinsed

3 cups boiling spring or filtered water

1/2 cup diced onion, carrot, and celery

1/2 cup yellow cornmeal, plus some more for dredging

Heat oil in a pot over medium heat. Add ginger, pinch of salt and cook 2-3 minutes. Remove ginger from oil and add millet and cook, stirring, until the millet is coated with oil. Carefully add boiling water, season lightly with salt to taste and reduce heat to low. Cover and simmer 35 minutes, add onion, carrot and celery, recover and simmer for another 5 minutes. Begin to form burgers.

Shape the millet mixture into thick patties. Dredge in cornmeal to coat. Heat about1/8 inch avocado oil in a skillet over medium heat. Fry patties until golden, about 3 minutes on each side. Remove from skillet and drain on paper towel to absorb excess oil. Serve as you would a regular burger.

Soft Rice With Barley (serves 4)

Ingredients

1 cup brown rice rinsed

1/4 cup barley, rinsed

6 cups spring water

1/8 tsp salt

1/2 cup walnuts, toasted

Umeboshi vinegar, to taste

1/4 cup scallions, chopped

1 sheet nori, cut into strips

In a pressure cooker, add brown rice, barley, and water. Soak overnight. Add salt and cover

Barley is the oldest known cultivated grain, comes in three forms, hulled, pearled, and hato mugi. The Hulled barley has the outer husk removed, keeping vitamin rich endosperm and germ layers intact. The pearled barley is not as nutritious, which is polished, removing both the endosperm and germ layers. Hato mugi (Job's tears) is wild grass with properties similar to barley.

Millet Croquettes

Millet has downward settling energy which supports digestion.

Ingredients (serves 6)

1 cup millet

3 cups spring water

1/2 cup pumpkin seeds, toasted

1/2 bunch scallions, minced

1/2 bunch parsley, minced

1 small carrot, finely grated

Shoyu, to taste

1/4 cup safflower oil

Parsley Almond Curry Sauce

Parsley Almond Curry Sauce

This sauce is great to supplement with vegetables and veggie burgers. Blend 1/4 cup almond butter, 1 TBSP curry paste, 1 1/2 TBSP shoyu and 1/4 cup of chopped parsley with 1/4 cup water. Curry paste: heat 2 TBSP of curry powder with 1 tsp extra virgin olive oil. You can try various nut butters and herbs for variations.

In a saucepan, dry roast millet over medium heat, stirring constantly, approximately 5-6 minutes. Remove from heat, add water and soak overnight.

Bring to boil lower heat, and simmer, covered, approximately 30 minutes. Transfer to a bowl.

Grind pumpkin seeds in a food processor. Add seeds, scallions, parsley, and carrot to millet. Mix and season with shoyu.

Form millet into croquettes. Heat oil in skillet and pain fry croquettes until browned on each side.

Serve with the Parsley Almond Curry Sauce.

Fried Rice Balls

This will increase your stamina.

4 sheets nori sea vegetable, pre toasted

4 cups brown rice

8 tsp tahini paste

4 TBSP sesame seeds (brown or black)

Extra Virgin Olive Oil or sesame oil for frying

Dipping sauce

2 tbsp shoyu

2 tbsp water

1 tbsp brown rice vinegar

1 tsp ginger, finely grated

2 tbsp daikon, finely grated

The nori sheets should be toasted, if not toasted, over a low flame, drag over the fire until the nori become lighter in color. Cut into quarters with a scissor and lay them out on dry surface.

Wet your hands, mold a handful of the rice mixture to form a ball (wetting hands frequently will help the rice from sticking to your hands).

Lay the ball of the rice onto the sheet of nori, spread the ball with 1 tsp tahini and sprinkle on sesame seeds. Place another sheet of nori on top and shape so the corners are between the corners of the lower sheet. Pick up the rice ball and squeeze so that nori sticks to the rice.

Add sufficient oil to coat the bottom of the cast iron skillet and heat gently. Add the rice balls and fry turning them gently until the nori is brown all over. Place a paper towel next to the pan and when done frying the rice balls, place on top to absorb the excess oil.

Mix all the dipping sauce ingredients together and divide between 4 individual small dishes. Serve the rice balls with the sauce. Enjoy.

Millet-Corn Loaf

5-6 servings

1 small onion, finely diced

1 small carrot, finely diced

1 ear of fresh corn, kernels removed, or frozen corn is ok

1 1/2 cup millet, rinsed well

6 cups filtered water

Sea salt

2-3 green onions, thinly sliced

2 TBSP umeboshi vinegar

3 TBSP sesame tahini

In a heavy pot, place diced onion, carrot, corn, and millet. Add water and a pinch of salt. Cover and bring to a boil over medium heat. Reduce heat and simmer 25-30 minutes. Season lightly with salt and simmer 5 minutes. Stir in the green onions and remove from the heat.

Preheat oven to 350F, lightly oil the loaf pan and set aside. Whisk together vinegar and tahini and stir into cooked millet mixture. Press mixture into prepared pan and bake, uncovered, 15 minutes. Allow to cool slightly before slicing. Slice and serve.

Millet Tofu Stew

Makes 4-5 servings

1 cup millet

1 cup cubed winter squash

1/2 cup small cubes extra-firm tofu

5 cups filtered water

1 tsp barley miso

1-2 green onions, thinly sliced

Rinse millet thoroughly.

Layer squash and tofu in a heavy pot and top with millet. Gently add water, cover and bring to a boil over medium heat. Reduce heat and simmer until liquid is absorbed and millet has a creamy texture, about 30 minutes. Dissolve miso in a small amount of warm water and gently stir into millet. Simmer 3-4 minutes and remove from heat and stir. Serve hot, garnish with green onions.

Maki Rolls

4-5 servings

2 sheets toasted sushi nori

1 cup cooked brown rice

2-3 stir fried carrot match sticks

Fresh Sauerkraut

Steam spinach

Pickled ginger or dipping sauce (soy sauce, water, ginger and diced green onion)

On the bamboo sushi mat, place the nori on the mat. Press the rice flat over the nori sheet, making sure that the rice covers the nori end to end, rice should be about 1/4 inch thick. Place the carrots, spinach, sauerkraut and then using the mat as a guide, roll the nori maki, jelly roll style. Remember, you are pressing the nori rice into a roll, once the bamboo mat is rolled and the nori sealed, remove the mat. With a sharp, wet knife, cut into 8 rounds, each about 1 inch thick. Place on a serving platter and serve with ginger.

Special Rice

Makes 3-4 servings

1 1/2 cups brown basmati rice, rinsed, soaked for 1 hour and drained.

1/2 cup wild rice, rinsed

2 1/2 cups filtered water

sea salt

1/4 cup orange juice

1/2 cup dried currants

2 tangerines

2 TBSP pine nuts

2-3 TBSP extra virgin olive oil.

2 TBSP sweet brown rice vinegar

Combine both rice in a pressure cooker with water and bring to a boil, add salt and seal the lid and bring to a full pressure. Place on low heat and cook 25 minutes. Turn off heat and allow pressure cooker to stand undisturbed for another 25 minutes.

In the meantime, heat the orange juice in a small saucepan until hot and pour over the currants to soften them. Peel and section the tangerine, being careful to remove all threads to prevent the bitter taste. Lightly toast the pine nuts in a dry skillet, approximately 2-3 minutes and set aside.

Open the pressure cooker and stir in the currants and juice, tangerine segments, olive oil, and rice vinegar. Stir well and transfer to a serving bowl and add the pine nuts right before serving and enjoy!

Barley with vegetables

Makes 4-5 servings

2 (1 inch) pieces kombu

2 cups whole barley, rinsed and soaked 6-8 hours and drained

6 cups filtered water

sea salt

1 onion finely diced

1/2 cup 1/2 inch cubes turnip

1 small carrot, cut into 1/2 inch cubes

1/2 cup thinly sliced fresh burdock

2-3 dried shiitake mushrooms, soaked and thinly sliced

2 stalks celery thinly sliced

Place kombu in a heavy pot and add barley and water. Cover and bring to a boil over medium heat then lower heat, add salt and simmer on low for approximately 40 minutes. Layer vegetables, except celery, on top of barley. Cover pot and simmer until the barley is creamy and vegetables are soft, about 40-45 minutes. Stir in celery and transfer to a serving bowl, serve hot.

Buckwheat Pancakes

Buckwheat is high in magnesium and antioxidants, which is very good for cardiovascular health.

Serves 4

1 cup Buckwheat flour

1/2 cup spelt flour

1 tsp ground cinnamon

1/8 teaspoon salt

3 TBSP safflower oil

1 1/2 cups almond milk

In a large bowl, mix dry ingredients together. Mix the wet ingredients in a separate bowl. Pour the wet ingredients into dry ingredients and mix. Cover the bowl with moist towel, and let batter sit overnight at room temperature.

Brush the bottom of skillet with safflower oil and heat over medium heat. Spread the batter onto the skillet making a pancake. When the bottom side gets browned, flip over and cook until the second side is browned. When cooked, remove to a plate, continue with the remaining batter.

Serve with honey or maple syrup.

Quinoa and pumpkin seed pilaf

Quinoa is an alkalizing grain which is very nutritious.

1 tsp olive oil

1/2 cup onion, diced

1/2 cup carrot, diced

1/4 cup celery, diced

1 cup quinoa, rinsed

2 cups water or vegetable broth

1/8 tsp salt

1/4 cup fresh parsley, finely chopped

1 tsp umeboshi paste

1/4 cup pumpkin seeds, toasted

1 tsp tahini

1/2 tsp shoyu

Lemon juice to taste

In a skillet, heat oil and saute onion, carrot, and celery until onion is translucent.

In a saucepan, dry roast quinoa over low flame for 5 minutes until fragrant.

Add water or broth, onion, carrot, celery, and salt. Bring to boil, lower heat, and simmer, covered for 20 minutes.

Mix in the remaining ingredients except for the lemon juice.

Add lemon juice to taste.

Brown Rice Burgers

Great way to prepare left over grain.

Serves 12

2 cups brown rice rinsed

4 cups filtered water

1/2 tsp salt

1 TBSP tahini

3 medium scallions, finely sliced

2 TBSP umeboshi paste

1/4 cup safflower oil

3 TBSP tamari, optional

Soak the brown rice over night in water, add water and salt and bring to a boil, lower heat and let simmer for 50 minutes.

Let the rice cool and stir in tahini and scallions. Wet hands and shape into balls. Dig a hole inside each one and add 1/4 tsp umeboshi paste. Flatten and shape into burgers.

Heat the oil in the skillet and pan fry each burger until browned on each side.

Serve

Mushroom Polenta Burgers

Serves 4

1 tsp olive oil

1/2 cup onion, minced

1 clove garlic, crushed

1/2 cup fresh shiitakes, minced

1 teaspoon fresh sage, chopped

1 tsp fresh rosemary, chopped

5 cups water

2 cups cornmeal

1/4 tsp salt

1/4 cup safflower oil

In a skillet, heat olive oil and sauté onion and garlic until translucent. Add the mushrooms, sage, and rosemary, and saute until mushrooms are cooked through.

In a saucepan, bring water to boil. Add cornmeal, mushroom and onion mixture, and salt. Lower the heat and continue stirring until all water is absorbed.

Pour polenta into baking pan, let it cool in the refrigerator.

Cut out the circles, using cookie cutter or large glass jar.

Heat safflower oil in skillet and pan fry burgers until browned on both sides.

Millet, quinoa pilaf with Burdock

Burdock adds the Yin (downward) energy, strengthens the kidney and the large intestine.

Serves 8

3/4 cup millet, rinsed

3 3/4 cups spring water

1/2 cup burdock, cut into matchsticks

2 tsp sesame oil

1/2 cup onion, diced

1/2 cup carrot, cut into matchsticks

1/2 cup red quinoa, rinsed

1/4 tsp salt

1/4 cup toasted walnuts, chopped

1/4 cup parsley, minced

Dry roast millet in saucepan until fragrant. Add water and soak overnight.

In a saucepan, sauté burdock in oil until soft, about 5 minutes. Add the onions and carrot and sauté until onion is translucent.

Bring millet and water to boil, lower heat and simmer for 10 minutes

Add the quinoa, vegetables, and salt. Bring to boil, lower heat, and simmer, covered 20 more minutes.

Mix walnuts into the dish, garnish with parsley.

Mediterranean Brown Rice Salad

Serves 4

2 cups brown rice, cooked

1/2 cup black pitted olives, chopped

1/4 cup carrots, grated

1 batch basil lemon mustard vinaigrette

6 large lettuce leaves, romaine

1/4 cup pine nuts, toasted

Basil Lemon Mustard Vinaigrette

1/3 cup fresh basil

1 TBSP Dijon mustard

1/2 cup olive oil

3 TBSP Tahini

2 cloves garlic, minced

2 TBSP lemon juice

Shoyu to taste

In a blender or food processor, mix all ingredients together, except shoyu. Season with Shoyu to taste.

Mix brown rice, olives, and carrots together.

Add the vinaigrette and mix, roll in the lettuce leaves with pine nuts.

Beans

Beans are high in proteins, great source of fiber and nutrients. Most beans are hard and need to be soaked overnight to improve digestibility. To remove the discomfort of excess gas, which they are known for, throw away the soaking water, except when soaking aduki beans and black soybeans because in Japan, this soaked water is known to be medicinal.

To cook beans, bring them to a boil and skim off the gas causing foam that rises to the top. Cooking beans with stamp sized bay leaf to add minerals and soften the beans, making a more balanced digestible dish. Season the beans when they are about 80% cooked with sea salt or soy sauce. Cooked beans can safely be used for 1-2 days.

Black soybeans with Chestnuts

Black soybeans increase blood circulation, detoxifies, and supports kidney health.

Serves 6

1 cup black soybeans, soaked in 4 cups water

1/4 cup dried chestnuts, soaked

1 piece of kombu, soaked

Shoyu to taste

Place beans and soaking water in pressure cooker. Bring to a boil, skim off any foam. Add the chestnuts and kombu. Cover, bring to pressure, lower the heat and pressure cook for 50 minutes.

Season with shoyu to taste.

Black eyed pea burgers

Serves 6

1 cup black eyed peas, soaked

Spring water as needed

1 piece of kombu, soaked

1 TBSP umeboshi paste

2 medium scallions, chopped

1/4 cup safflower oil

Rinse beans and place in a pressure cooker. Add enough water to cover beans by 1". Bring to a boil, and skim off any foam. Add the kombu, cover and bring to pressure, lower the heat, and pressure cook for 20 minutes (or simmer on stove for 1 hour).

Mash beans, and season with umeboshi paste, then add scallions

Form bean puree into 6-8 patties. Place in refrigerator to firm, in a skillet, pan fry patties in oil until browned on both sides.

Garbanzo Beans in Mushroom Gravy

chickpeas or garbanzo beans supports the digestion. Mushrooms strengthen liver function, the white mushrooms are rich in antioxidants and are ant carcinogenic.

Serves 6

11/2 cups garbanzo beans, soaked

Spring water, as needed, and 21/2 cups

1 piece kombu soaked

1 medium onion, diced

1 tsp olive oil

12 white button mushrooms, sliced

2 TBSP mirin (optional)

1/2 cup shoyu

2 TBSP kuzu

Drain beans and place in pressure cooker. Add enough water to cover beans by 1 inch. Bring to a boil and remove any foam, and the kombu and cover, bring to pressure, lower the heat and cook for 30 minutes.

Saute onion in oil until translucent. Add mushrooms and saute until cooked through. Add 2 cups water, mirin, and shoyu. Simmer for about a minute. Dissolve the kuzu in 1/2 cup water and add the kuzu mixture to onions and simmer 2 minutes and adjust the seasoning to taste.

Once the beans are cooked, drain, and add to the mushroom gravy and serve.

Garlic Garbanzo Beans

Serves 6

1 cup garbanzo beans, soaked

Spring water as needed

1 piece of kombu, soakes

2 cloves garlic, roasted

1/4 cup sesame seeds, toasted

1/1/2 TBSP umeboshi vinegar

1/4 cup olive oil

2 medium scallions, chopped

1/4 cup dill, chopped

Lemon juice to taste

Drain garbanzo beans and place in pressure cooker, add water to cover beans by an inch. Bring to boil and remove foam. Add kombu and cover pressure cooker. Bring to pressure, lower heat, and pressure cook for 25 minutes. Drain the beans.

Mince the garlic, grind the toasted sesame seeds into powder. Season beans with umeboshi vinegar, olive oil, scallions, garlic, ground sesame seeds, dill, and lemon juice. Marinate beans overnight for best flavor before serving.

Lima beans and corn

Serves 6

1 cup lima beans, soaked

Spring water, as needed

1 piece kombu soaked

3 cups fresh corn kernels

1 tsp olive oil

2 tsp sweet white miso

1/2 cup chives chopped

Drain beans. Place beans in a sauce pan and cover with water by about an inch. Bring to a boil and remove foam. Add kombu, lower heat, and simmer for 1 1/2 hours or until tender, adding more water if needed.

Add corn, olive oil, and sweet white miso and simmer for 5 minutes. Garnish with chives and serve.

Vegetables

Our current culture relies on animal foods as the mainstay of most meals. I believe it is due to the Atkins movement in recommending high protein meals and decided to put a label on the carbohydrates such as the whole grains and breads and declared it as forbidden. We need to understand that the consumption of animal products are very taxing on our organ systems. The assimilation of the foods, the animal foods require so much exertion from our various organs vs the vegetable foods are so easily digested and absorbed.

So let's make a commitment together to incorporate more vegetables in our foods. I highly recommend researching the local farmers and support them. While I recommend eating organic, the FDA standards are at times impossible for the small farmers to adhere to. The "organic" certification is usually too expensive for the small local farmers, however, they are still complying with the "organic" standards, just can't afford the certification label so why not support them? In my community, we have CSA (community sustained agriculture) where a group of people in the community will pay for the share of the vegetable crops for a season. This way we get local, and organic produce while supporting our farmers. For me, it's been nice to get produce this way and know exactly where my food comes from.

Get in the habit of selecting variety of vegetables and combining the root vegetables such as carrots, turnips, parsnips, burdock, rutabaga, ground vegetables such as squash, onion, broccoli, cabbage, brussels sprouts, cauliflower, and Chinese cabbage. Incorporate the dark greens such as kale, collards, mustards, watercress, escarole, arugula, lettuces, bok choy, rapini, and some herbs and grasses and just explore your options. Once you start to know the vegetables, you will be surprised at how much choices you have.

Caveats

While vegetables are generally all good for you, here are the tips on how to combine your vegetables for optimal health:

- Spinach, chard, parsley, and purslane are rich sources of oxalic acid a compound known to inhibit the body to absorb calcium efficiently. If you are struggling with bone loss and osteoporosis, keep these to a minimum. However, these vegetables can be neutralized by combining with other vegetables.

- The nightshade family of vegetables, including tomatoes, potatoes, bell peppers and egg plant all contain mildly toxic acids that affect people with arthritis by causing further inflammation. Keep in mind that these acids are somewhat neutralized by cooking, marinating, drying, juicing, or roasting. However, if you have acute symptoms of arthritis, this minute amount can still cause irritation so avoid them. These vegetables are so delicious, high in vitamins and nutrients, it would be sad to give them up.

- Then there are the tropical vegetables and fruit. They are grown in hot climates and nature designed them to cool the bodies in hot weather. They include: oranges, grapefruit, papaya, banana, mango, yucca, plantain, and other tropical treats can leave us feeling too cold. They are also rich in simple sugars which can wreak havoc on our immune system. They also have a acidifying effect in the body, however, one need not avoid completely, you can still enjoy by food combining.

Storing vegetables

It is best to store your vegetables in cotton or plastic bags. I don't recommend that you wash your vegetables before storing, if you do wash them, dry them best as you can and wrap them in paper towel before putting into a ziploc bag.

Cooking vegetables

Cooking vegetables are a way to make them more digestible so that we can assimilate them with ease.

Boiling/Blanching

Boiling is a quick and efficient way to produce firm, full bodied flavors with vibrant colors while maintaining the nutrients in the vegetables. Boiling the vegetables also employs a good bit of moisture, and as a result nourishes the skin, making it soft and resilient.

It is best to use a deep pot with plenty of water, cook the vegetables in small amounts so as not to lose the boil. It is ideal to use a pinch of salt in the water which will help the vegetables to retain the nutrients.

Remember, boiled and blanched vegetables continue to cook even after you remove from the heat, so to keep them from cooking, I recommend that you plunge them in cold water to cool.

Steaming

Steaming is cooking in hot steam produced by boiling a small amount of water. Unlike boiling, the vegetables are cooked on racks above the water. Collapsible stainless steel racks or bamboo steamers are most commonly used.

Bring the water to a high boil before adding the vegetables and cover the pot tightly while cooking. It is best when the vegetables are arranged in a single layer. This cooking method imparts great vitality into the vegetables as they are cooked over high heat, very quickly, with very little moisture.

Stewing/Braising

Braising is slow simmering in a small amount of stock or some other liquid, like oil. Braising is generally cooking one vegetable vs the stewing is combination of several vegetables simmering in their own juice. This cooking method results in very sweet tasting vegetables.

Sautéing

The French word for jump or leap is sauté. To saute, heat a small amount of oil in a skillet; the hot oil sears the skin of the vegetable, allowing it to cook, but sealing in the nutrients and flavor. It is important to add the vegetables slowly, if the heat reduces too much, it would steam rather than sautéing them. To make sure you don't end up with limp vegetables, make sure to dry them before sautéing, and stir frequently to prevent from sticking.

Baking and Roasting

This cooking method may take longer to cook, but it requires no work during the cooking process. Winter squash, brussels sprouts, parsnips, leeks, celery, cauliflower, zucchini, yellow squash, and asparagus are all perfect for this method of cooking. All you have to do is cut the vegetables in desired size and sprinkle with a bit of sea salt to seal in the moisture and bring out the flavor of the vegetable.

Broiling/Grilling

Broiling and grilling consist of cooking vegetables over high heat until the outside areas are lightly seared and insides are tender. The vegetables can be marinated with just sea salt and pepper and extra virgin olive oil.

Pickling

Vegetables do really well with this technique. It's used in Asia a lot more than in the west. Pickled foods aid in the digestion of our foods as well, this is thanks to the fermentation process that uses the bacteria to convert the sweetness into the lactic acid that aids in the digestive process. Pickling also enhances the vitamins B and C.

Sea Vegetables

Sea vegetables have been used in the east for centuries. Sea vegetables are both nutritious and detoxifying. They contain ample amount of chlorophyll, which aids in the production of hemoglobin for red blood cell production. In its traditional for a woman who just had a baby to consume sea weed soup for days to clear the blood. I too had to succumb to this tradition as both my mother in law and my mother were adamant about this intake after I delivered my boys.

Here are the recipes to enjoy.

Arame with Corn, green beans, and Onions

Arame stabilizes blood pressure and blood sugar levels. Feel free to explore different vegetables such as beets, carrots, and edamame.

Serves 4

1 medium red onions, cut into half moons

1 tsp sesame oil

1 cup arame, rinsed

1/2 cup green beans

1/2 cup fresh corn off the cob or frozen corn

Spring water as needed

1 1/2 tsp tamari

Brown rice vinegar to taste

1 TBSP fresh Dill, chopped.

In a skillet, saute onion in oil until translucent. Layer arame on top of onions, green beans, and corn. Add the water half way up to the top of the vegetables. Bring to boil, lower heat and simmer for 20 minutes.

Season with tamari, stir, and continue to cook , uncovered until all liquid is evaporated.

Season to taste with brown rice vinegar. Garnish with dill and leave covered for 2 minutes and serve.

Wild Nori Fried Rice

NOri is rich in iron, vitamins, and minerals. Nourishes the circulatory system and help to prevent hardening of the arteries. Nori enriches and cleanses the blood, which is detoxifying. It is also antibiotic and aids in tissue healing.

Serves 6

1/2 cup wild nori

1 cup red onion diced

2 cloves garlic, crushed

1 TBSP olive oil

1/2 tsp sesame oil

1 medium carrot, cut into match sticks

1/2 cup celery diced

1/2 cup broccoli, chopped

3 cups cooked brown rice

4 TBSP water

3 TBSP shoyu

2 medium scallions sliced

Gomashio to taste

Toast wild nori in the oven at 300 degrees F for 5-8 minutes, turning occasionally, until crisp. Crumble or cut into flakes.

In a wok or heavy skillet, saute onion and garlic in live and sesame oil for 5-7 minutes and add carrots and celery, saute for another 5-7 minutes. Add the cooked rice, water, and shoyu and stir for 2 minutes. Taste and adjust seasonings. Add the nori and stir.

Garnish with scallions and gomashio and serve.

Authentic Vegetable Salad (Some of the sea ingredients may be only available at the Asian grocery store)

Serves 4

1/2 cup snow pea pods

Spring water as needed

Pinch sea salt

1/2 cup carrots, cut into matchsticks

1/2 cup sea palm (may be hard to find)

1/2 cup sea whip fronds (may be hard to find)

1 TBSP shoyu

4 TBSP sweet brown rice

1 TBSP toasted sesame oil

Toasted walnuts, chopped, optional

Orange zest, optional

Remove the ends and strings from snow pea pods. Bring one pot of water to boil and add a pinch of sea salt. Boil carrots fro 2-3 minutes and remove with a slotted spoon. Boil pea pods 1-2 minutes and remove with a slotted spoon. Chop the sea vegetables at a desired length. Place all ingredients in a mixing bowl.

Add sweet brown rice vinegar, shoyu, and sesame oil and stir. Garnish with toasted chopped walnuts and oranges zest.

Baked Brussels Sprouts and Shallots

This is absolutely delicious.

Serves 4-5

2-3 cups fresh brussels sprouts, trimmed and left whole

3-4 shallots halved

2 or 3 cloves fresh garlic, finely minced

Sea salt

215

2 TBSP extra virgin olive oil or coconut oil

2 TBSP balsamic vinegar

Preheat oven to 375 F

Cut a slight cross through each brussels sprouts to ensure cooking through. In a baking pan or casserole dish, arrange the Brussels sprouts and shallots, avoiding overlap. Sprinkle generously with garlic, shake sea salt sparingly and coat with olive oil and balsamic vinegar.

Cover the casserole or the baking pan with foil and bake 40-45 minutes. Remove the cover and bake until vegetables are lightly browned. Gently toss before serving and enjoy.....

Delectable Mashed Cauliflower

Serves 3-4

1 Head cauliflower broken into florets

1/8 cup unsweetened almond or coconut milk

3 TBSP vegetarian buttery spread

Sea salt

Cracked black pepper

Small bunch chives, finely minced

Steam the cauliflower by placing them on the steam basket in a pot, cook until cooked (fork tender), approximately 11-12 minutes.

Preheat the oven to 325F. Lightly oil the baking dish and set aside. Transfer the cauliflower to the food processor or the blender. Add the coconut or almond milk, spread, salt and pepper and puree until soft. Spoon into prepared baking dish and bake uncovered for approximately 8 minutes until bubbly. Fold in the chives and serve hot.

Guacamole

Avocados are alkalizing, great source of vitamins and minerals, and good source of healthy fat. Enjoy without guilt.

Serves 3-4

2 ripe avocados, halved and seed removed

1/2 red onion, finely minced

2 Serrano chiles, seeded, ribs removed and finely minced

2 TBSP finely minced cilantro

1/4 cup fresh or frozen corn kernels

1-2 TBSP fresh lemon juice

Sea salt

Cracked black pepper

1/2 ripe tomato, seeded and chopped

Place the avocados into a bowl, using a fork, mash the avocados until smooth. Fold in the onion, chiles, cilantro, corn, and lemon juice. Mix in salt and pepper to taste. Gently add the tomato, chill for at least an hour before serving to allow the flavors to flourish.

Stuffed Zucchini

Makes 4 servings

2 large zucchini, split lengthwise, scoop out the flesh

(above flesh mashed and save)

Extra virgin olive oil

2 cloves fresh garlic, finely minced

1 onion diced

Sea salt

Pinch of red pepper flakes if desired

2 stalks celery, cut into small dice

1/2 cup diced vegan mozzarella cheese alternative or the raw milk derivative (organic mozzarella is acceptable)

Whole wheat bread crumbs

2 cups organic tomato sauce

Preheat oven to 375F, lightly oil the baking dish. Place a small amount of oil, garlic and onion in a skillet over medium heat. Add a pinch of salt when the onion begins to sizzle and sauté for 3-4 minutes. In another skillet, place a small amount of oil, celery and mashed zucchini over medium heat, when the contents begins sizzle, add pinch of salt and sauté for 2 minutes. Stir in the sautéed onions and garlic and combine and stir. Remove from heat and add the cheese, fold in the bread crumbs to hold the mixture together as stuffing (approximately 1/2 cup to 1 cup).

Spoon the mixture into the zucchini halves, spoon the tomato sauce on top and bake uncovered until the filling is set, approximately 30 minutes. Serve hot and enjoy....

Ratatouille

4 Servings

3 TBSP Extra Virgin Olive Oil

3 cloves fresh garlic, finely minced

2 tsp dried basil

1 eggplant, cut into 1/2 inch cubes, soaked in salted water 1 hour and drained

Sea salt

1 cup extra firm tofu, finely crumbled

2 tsp white miso

2 zucchini, thinly sliced on the diagonal

1 large red onion, sliced into thin rings

2 cups thinly sliced cremini mushrooms

1 red bell pepper, roasted over a flame, peeled, seeded and thinly sliced

2 large, ripe tomatoes, coarsely chopped

Preheat oven to 350F, oil a 2 quart casserole with 1 TBSP of the oil and set aside.

Place remaining oil, garlic and basil in a skillet over medium heat. Sauté garlic until lightly browned. Stir in eggplant, sauté until eggplant is soft, about 10 minutes. Season lightly with salt and sauté 1 minute.

Spread eggplant evenly over the bottom of prepared casserole. Mix crumbled tofu and miso together and sprinkle a few TBSP of the tofu mixture over the eggplant. Layer the zucchini over the tofu sprinkle with a few TBSP of the tofu mixture. Continue layering in this order; onion, tofu, mixture mushrooms, tofu mixture, bell pepper, tofu and finally top with tomatoes. Bake uncovered for 45 minutes, remove from the oven and allow to stand 10 minutes before serving.

Portobello Burgers

6 servings

Portobello mushrooms have a "meaty" texture, perfect as a burger.

Onion Topping

Extra Virgin Olive Oil

2-3 cloves fresh garlic, thinly sliced

5-6 red onions, thin half moon slices

Sea salt

Mirin or white wine

Generous pinch crushed red pepper flakes

Juice of 1/2 lemon

2-3 TBSP extra virgin olive oil or avocado oil, plus extra for brushing

1 TBSP balsamic vinegar

Pinch of red pepper flakes

Sea salt

6 portobello mushrooms, stems removed, gills intact, brushed free of dirt

6 whole grain burger buns

Ketchup (organic) Organic Mustard (optional)

6 leaves romaine lettuce

1-2 ripe tomatoes, sliced into rings

6-8 TBSP alfalfa sprouts

Make onion topping: Place a small amount of oil, garlic, and onions in a deep skillet over medium heat, add a pinch of salt when it comes to a sizzle. Also add in the mirin and red pepper flakes and sauté 3-4 minutes. Season lightly with salt and cook, stirring occasionally until the onions caramelize as long as 25 minutes. Remove from the heat, stir in lemon juice and set aside.

Preheat the grill to hot or warm a lightly oiled grill pan over a medium heat. Whisk together olive oil, vinegar, red pepper flakes and a generous pinch of salt. Rub each mushroom thoroughly with the oil mixture and grill on both sides until tender and lightly browned 5-6 minutes each side.

To assemble the burgers, brush one side of each slice of the rolls lightly with oil and grill, oil side down, until lightly browned, about 2 minutes. Lay the bread slices, grilled side up, on a dry work surface. Spread the ketchup and mustard if you are using and lay a lettuce leaf and tomato slice on 6 slice on 6 halves of the rolls. Lay the portobello on top of the lettuce, mound the onion topping and top with sprouts, place the top of buns and serve.

Roasted Squash and Mushrooms

4 Servings

6 TBSP extra virgin olive oil

1 tsp sea salt

4 cups cubed unpeeled delicate or butternut squash

4 cups mixed mushrooms (cremini, shiitake, oyster), stemmed, halved

Juice of 1/2 fresh lemon

Preheat oven to 425F. Place oil, salt, squash and mushrooms in a mixing bowl and toss to coat. Spread over a baking pan avoiding overlap. Bake uncovered 25-35 minutes until vegetables are tender. Remove from oven and drizzle with lemon juice, serve hot and enjoy.....

Zucchini Fettuccini with Marinara

Serves 4-6

1-2 pounds plum tomatoes, quartered

1 cup packed fresh basil leaves, plus some for garnish

1/2 cup dry packed sun dried tomatoes, softened in warm water and chopped

4 TBSP extra virgin olive oil

1 tsp brown rice syrup

1 shallot, minced

sea salt

cracked black pepper

3 zucchini, ends trimmed

1 summer squash, ends trimmed

1 red or orange bell pepper, halved and seeded

8 oz vegan mozzarella cheese alternative or organic mozzarella, grated

1 cup coarsely chopped hazelnuts

Place tomatoes, basil, sun-dried tomatoes 3 TBSP of the oil, rice syrup, shallot and salt and pepper to taste in a food processor and process until mixture resembles a fine salsa. Using a sharp vegetable peeler, pare zucchini and summer squash on all sides. Discard soft, seeded centers.

Using a sharp knife, slice bell pepper into very thin strips. Combine the squash, zucchini and bell pepper in a mixing bowl. Stir in tomato mixture and adjust seasonings to your taste, fold in the cheese and hazelnuts and stir gently to combine ingredients. Serve garnished with basil sprigs.

Roasted Vegetables

Serves 4-6

This is a simple way to serve the vegetables.

1 bay leaf

2 cups button mushrooms, brushed clean and left whole

2 cups small brussels sprouts, trimmed and left whole

2 parsnips, cut into large, irregular chunks

2 leeks, rinsed well and cut into 2 inch pieces

2 cups 1 inch daikon chunks

Soy sauce

Extra virgin olive oil

Reduced balsamic vinegar

2 tsp fresh lemon juice

Preheat oven to 375F, place bay leaf on the bottom of a shallow baking dish to help tenderize and sweeten vegetables. Arrange the vegetables and sprinkle lightly with soy sauce and oil, coating the vegetables well. Cover the baking dish and bake about 1 hour, until vegetables are tender. Remove the cover, stir in a light sprinkling of reduced balsamic vinegar. Toss gently with lemon juice and remove bay leaf before serving.

Green Beans Vinaigrette

Serves 5-6

1 pound green beans

Spring water

VINAIGRETTE

1 TBSP extra virgin olive oil

2 cloves fresh garlic, thinly sliced

Juices of 1 lemon

2-3 TBSP prepared stone ground mustard

1 TBSP brown rice vinegar

1 TBSP Umeboshi vinegar

1 TBSP brown rice syrup

Generous pinch dried rosemary

Slivered almonds, lightly pan toasted for garnish

Remove bean tips and thinly slice beans on the diagonal, making long, thin slivers. Bring water to a boil in a pot. Add beans and cook until tender and bright green, about 3 minutes. Drain the beans and set aside to cool.

Prepare the vinaigrette: Heat olive oil in a small skillet over medium heat. Add garlic and cook until brown, about 3 minutes. Skim garlic from the oil and discard. Whisk together the lemon juice, mustard, salt to taste, vinegars, rice syrup, rosemary to taste and garlic-flavored oil. Whisk until well emulsified. Toss the dressing with the cooked beans and serve warm or chilled, garnished with the almonds.

Sautéed Dark Greens with Ginger

Serves 3-4

2 TBSP avocado oil

6-7 slices fresh ginger, cut into fine matchsticks

1 bunch leafy greens (kale or collards) cleaned and finely chopped

Soy sauce

1-2 tsp fresh ginger juice

Dark sesame oil for finishing

Heat oil in a deep skillet over medium heat. Add ginger and cook 1-2 minutes. Add greens and sprinkle lightly with soy sauce. Cook until bright green and tender, but not mushy, 2-3 minutes. If you like the ginger flavor, you can also add ginger extract at the end of cooking to intensify the flavor. Transfer to a serving bowl, drizzle lightly with sesame oil to taste and serve.

Green Rolls

Serves 4-5

Spring water

3-4 carrot sticks

7-8 leaves Chinese cabbage, rinsed and left whole

1 bunch collard greens, rinsed and stems removed

1 bunch watercress, rinsed and left whole

Black sesame seeds, toasted for garnish

Bring a pot of water to a boil and separately boil each vegetable in the order listed above. Cook each until just crisp, approximately 1-3 minutes each. Lay on plates to cool.

To assemble the rolls, place 2-3 collard leaves on a bamboo sushi mat or dish towel. Top with 2-3 cabbage leaves, then place a thick strip of watercress and 1 carrot stick. Roll using the mat or the towel as a guide. When completely rolled, squeeze gently to seal the roll. Then slice into 1 inch thick rounds, arrange on a serving platter and sprinkle the tops of the rolls with black sesame seeds.

Onion Muffins

I love onions in anything...loaded with phytochemicals, chromium to help control the blood sugar, and rich in Vit C for improved immunity, what's not to love?

4-5 servings

PASTRY

1 cup whole wheat pastry flour

Pinch of sea salt

Avocado Oil

Cold Spring water

1 tsp avocado oil

2-3 medium onions finely diced

Sea salt

2 tsp brown rice syrup

Prepare pastry

Whisk the flour and salt together into a bowl. Slowly add about 3 TBSP of oil, creating the consistency of wet sand. Slowly add the water, by the TBSP, while stirring with a wooden spoon, until the dough is soft in consistency. Gather the dough into a ball and set aside, cover with a damp towel.

Heat oil in a skillet over low heat. Add onions, a light sprinkling of salt and rice syrup and cook until soft, sweet and caramelized, about 1 hour, stirring frequently to avoid sticking.

When the onions are almost done, finish the crusts: Preheat oven to 350 F. Lightly oil a 12 cup muffin pan and set aside. On a lightly floured surface, thinly roll out the dough into about 12X9 inch rectangle. Cut the dough into about 3 inch rounds and press each one into a prepared muffin cup. Prick each crust in several places and fill each with cooked onions. Bake about 20 minutes, until the crusts are golden and the filling begins to set. Cool slightly before removing from the muffin cups. Best served with a hearty soup or a fresh salad. Enjoy.....

Sweet Glazed Onions

Serves 4

4 medium onions

Corn kernels cut from 1 ear of corn or 1 cup frozen corn

1/2 cup finely diced winter squash

1 carrot finely diced

1/2 cup whole wheat bread crumbs

Spring water

2 TBSP brown rice syrup

3-4 TBSP stone ground mustard

Generous dash of balsamic vinegar

Sea salt

Extra Virgin Olive Oil

Preheat oven to 375F. Peel the onions and cut each onion crosswise through the center into 2 equal halves. Remove the centers, leaving a bowl, dice the centers finely to use for filling.

Mix together the diced onion, corn, squash, carrot and enough bread crumbs and water to make a stuffing that holds together. Press the stuffing firmly into each onion bowl and arrange in a shallow baking dish so that onions fit together snugly. Pour tiny water into the dish.

Whisk together the rice syrup, mustard, vinegar and a generous pinch of salt. Spoon a little mustard sauce over each onion, reserving remaining sauce. Sprinkle each onion lightly with additional bread crumbs and drizzle with olive oil. Cover and bake 20-25 minutes. Remove cover, drizzle onions with remaining mustard mixture and a touch more oil and bake about 5 minutes. Serve warm and enjoy.....

Marinated Winter Greens

Serves 4

2-3 TBSP balsamic vinegar

Sea salt

2 cloves fresh garlic finely minced

1/4 cup extra virgin olive oil

4-5 button mushrooms, brushed clean and quartered

5-6 TBSP walnut pieces

1 bunch dark greens (kale, collards, broccoli, rapini), stems removed.

Whisk together vinegar, salt, garlic, and olive oil in a bowl. Add mushrooms and stir to coat. Allow to marinate 1 hour. Meanwhile, lightly pan toast the walnuts over medium heat, about 3 minutes. Finely chop and set aside.

Steam the greens until they are dark, rich green, approximately 3 minutes. Cut the greens into bite sized pieces. Just before serving, toss together the greens, walnuts, mushrooms, and remaining marinade and serve.

Chinese Vegetables

Serves 4-5

2-3 dried shiitake mushrooms, soaked until tender in warm water.

1 TBSP avocado oil

2-3 cloves of garlic, minced

1 onion, cut into thin half moon slices

Sea salt

1-2 carrots, cut into thin matchsticks

2-3 celery stalks, cut into thick diagonal

1 cup thin matchsticks of daikon

2-3 stalks of broccoli, cut into small florets

1 cup cauliflower, cut into small florets

4-5 snow peas, trimmed and left whole

CHINESE SAUCE

1-2 cups spring water

Soy sauce

1-2 tsp kuzu or arrowroot, dissolved in 1/4 cup cold water

1 TBSP brown rice vinegar

1 tsp dark sesame oil for finishing

Cut mushrooms into thin slices and simmer in soaking water 10 minutes to tenderize them.

Heat oil in a skillet or wok over medium heat, add garlic, onion, and pinch of salt and cook, stirring (approx 2-3 minutes). Drain and add mushrooms and a pinch of salt and cook, stirring 3-4 minutes. Add the carrots and pinch of salt, stir 2-3 minutes. Stir in the remaining vegetables except the snow peas, and cook approximately 3 minutes. Finally add the snow peas and sprinkle lightly with water, cover and steam approximately 3 minutes. Remove from heat.

SAUCE:

Heat water and soy sauce in a saucepan over medium heat. Stir in the dissolved kuzu and cook, stirring, until sauce is thick and clear, 3 minutes. Remove from heat and season with vinegar. Stir well and toss gently with cooked vegetables, drizzle with sesame oil and serve hot.

Green Beans with Herbs

Makes 4-5 servings

1 lbs fresh green beans, trimmed

2 TBSP extra virgin olive oil

2 TBSP balsamic vinegar

6-8 leaves fresh basil, minced

1/4 cup minced fresh flat leaf parsley

Sea salt

Juice of 1 lemon

Lemon slices or red pepper rings and fresh herb sprigs for garnish

Preheat oven 500F. Toss whole beans with oil, vinegar, a sprinkling of herbs and a pinch of salt. Spread on a baking sheet without overlapping beans too much. Oven roast, uncovered for about 10 minutes. Remove from the oven, toss with lemon juice and transfer to a serving bowl. Chill before serving. Garnish with lemon slices or red pepper rings and fresh herbs.

Roasted Onions

Makes 4 servings

6-8 onions, cut into thick wedges

2-3 cloves fresh garlic, finely minced

1 TBSP extra virgin olive oil

About 2 tsp spring water

Sea salt

Reduced balsamic vinegar

Juice of 1/4 lemon

Preheat oven to 375F, arrange onion wedges in a baking dish and sprinkle with garlic. Drizzle with oil, water, and light sprinkling of salt and a generous drizzle of reduced balsamic vinegar. Cover and bake about 45 minutes, remove the cover and bake about 30 minutes, until the onions are soft. Toss gently with lemon juice and transfer to a serving bowl, serve hot and enjoy.....

Vegetable Bean Stew

Serves 4-5

1 TBSP avocado oil

1 onion cut into large dice

Soy sauce

1 cup large dice winter squash

1 cup large dice white turnips

1 or 2 carrots, cut into large dice

1 or 2 parsnips, cut into large dice

2 TBSP whole wheat pastry flour

1 cup cooked kidney beans, drained

2-3 TBSP prepared stone-ground mustard

Fresh ginger juice

Spring water

2-3 stalks of broccoli cut into small florets for garnish

Preheat oven to 375F lightly oil a casserole dish and set aside

Heat oil in a skillet over medium heat. Add onion and a dash of soy sauce and cook until wilted. Add squash, turnips, carrots and parsnips and stir. Sprinkle lightly with soy sauce and cook a few more minutes and set aside.

Mix kidney beans, mustard, ginger juice and soy sauce in a large bowl. Fold in cooked vegetables, spoon into prepared casserole and sprinkle lightly with water. Cover and bake for 45 minutes. Remove the cover and bake for another 10 minutes.

While the stew is baking, steam broccoli, over boiling water until crisp tender, 5 minutes. When the casserole is done, remove from the oven and arrange broccoli around the edges of the casserole. Serve hot.

Noodle Dishes

With all the hype of "gluten free eating" I tried to stay off from the gluten, but truly, pasta, noodles, and breads are my favorite. I did my detoxification and found that I was not intolerant of gluten. I've experimented with introducing gluten back into my life and happy to report that this is not the issue for me. Many are not sensitive to gluten, if that's you, I hope you find the recipes useful. In Macrobiotics cooking noodle varieties can be prepared seasonally: udon (can be used all year), somen (used more in the summer), and soba (can be used all year). While the udon and the somen are made from wheat, soba is made from buckwheat flour which is more warming and yang. Keep in mind that although sobas are typically eaten in cool weather, soba can also be used in cold salad or cold broth in the summer to strengthen the kidneys.

I savor my noodle dishes, have learned to perfect some dishes and I'd like to share them here with you.

Cooking Tips

I am sure you've heard of "al dente" which means "chewy". Pasta should be firm but not undercooked and not mushy. Simply cook 1 minute less than what the package recommends and you are sure to get the "al dente" noodles. Salting the water helps to bring the water to a boil quicker, and helps to prevent the noodles from becoming too mushy.

In the east, we are taught to rinse our noodles, but our friends in Italy say to not rinse. My Italian friends say that this is because the flavor of the pasta sauce will be sealed better without the rinsing. However, the Asian dishes are different so we usually rinse our noodles. Who am I to argue with this?

Old Fashioned Spaghetti

Serves 4-5

Tomato Sauce

Extra Virgin Olive oil

1 small onion finely diced

3-4 cloves of garlic, finely minced

Sea salt

Pinch of dried oregano

1 (6 oz) organic tomato paste

Spring water

2 (28 oz) cans of organic diced tomatoes, undrained

1 carrot left whole

2 bay leaves

2-4 sprigs basil, leaves removed

Cracked black pepper

Organic Beef Meatballs (if desired)

1 cup organic ground beef

1/2 cup finely minced red onion

1/2 -2/3 cup fresh bread crumbs

1 tsp finely minced fresh basil

1/2 tsp dried oregano

1/2 tsp garlic powder

1/2 tsp sea salt

1/2 tsp black pepper

1/4 cup organic tomato paste

1 lb whole wheat spaghetti

Preheat oven to 375F (190C). Oil a baking sheet and set aside.

Prepare tomato sauce: Place a small amount of oil, onion and garlic in a soup pot over medium heat. When the onion begins to sizzle, add a pinch of salt and oregano and suate 2-3 minutes. Add tomato paste, 2 cans of water (tomato paste can) and stir until smooth. Add tomatoes with juice, a light seasoning of salt, carrot and bay leaves. Bring to a boil, reduce heat to low and cook, covered, 45 minutes stirring occasionally. Remove carrot and bay leaves; season to taste with salt and pepper; stir in basil and cook, uncovered, about 15 minutes.

Prepare meat balls: Combine all ingredients well and form into balls. Place on prepared baking sheet and bake 20 minutes, turning once, halfway through cooking.

Meanwhile, bring a pot of water to a boil, add a drizzle of oil and a pinch of salt. Cook spaghetti until just tender to the bite, about 10 minutes. Drain, do not rinse.

Mix balls gently into some of the sauce, toss spaghetti with sauce to coat and serve with the balls on top.

Korean Vermicelli Noodles (Jap Chae)

In Korea, it is customary to have this dish especially when it's a special occasion. I grew up with this dish, you can say that it's my comfort food. I top it off on a bed of brown short grain rice and eat with my Kimchee.

Makes 4 servings

6 oz very thin vermicelli noodles

1/2 cup soy sauce

3 TBSP sesame oil

3 TBSP brown rice syrup

2 cloves fresh garlic, minced

1 TBSP avocado oil

1 red onion, cut into thin half moon slices

2 carrots, fine matchstick pieces

1-2 cups button mushrooms, brushed free of dirt and thinly sliced

3 cups baby spinach or arugula

2 cups bean sprouts

Soak noodles in a bowl of warm water until softened, about 10 minutes. Drain in a colander. Bring a pot of water to a boil, add noodles, and cook 2 minutes. Drain well and rinse under cool water until cooked through.

Whist together the soy sauce, sesame oil, rice syrup, and garlic and set aside.

Heat the avocado oil in a deep skillet over medium heat. Add onions and saute 1 minute. Stir in carrots and saute 2 minutes. Stir in mushrooms and saute 3 minutes. Finally stir in the spinach and the bean sprouts and saute until just tender about 30 seconds. Stir in noodles and soy sauce mixture and cook, uncovered, until the liquid is absorbed, 3-4 minutes. Transfer cooked noodle mixture to a shallow platter and serve.

Soba Noodles with Ginger and Green Onions

This noodle dish, quickly sautéed with ginger and garlic, is delicious!

Serves 2-3

1 (8 oz) package soba noodles

1 TBSP light sesame oil

2 cloves fresh garlic, minced

2-3 dried shiitake mushrooms, soaked until tender and sliced

1-2 tsp freshly grated fresh ginger and juice

4-5 green onions, thinly sliced

1 tsp mirin

Soy sauce

1/4 cup minced fresh flat leaf parsley or mint for garnish

Cook noodles as directed on the package until tender, 8-10 minutes. Drain, rinse well and set aside

Heat oil in a skillet over medium heat. Add garlic and cook, stirring, until fragrant, about 2 minutes. Add mushrooms and cook, stirring, 3-4 minutes. Add grated ginger and juice to taste, green onions, mirin, a light seasoning of soy sauce and sesame seeds and cook, stirring, 2-3 minutes. Toss mixture with noodles and stir in parsley. Serve in bowl garnished with parsley.

Chinese Noodle Salad

This is a quick and easy dish packed with fresh vegetables....

Serves 2-3

Spring water

1/4 cup diced carrot

10-12 snow peas, cut into thin matchsticks

1/4 cup thin matchstick pieces of daikon

2-3 green onions, cut into thin diagonal pieces

3-4 slices fresh ginger, cut into thin matchsticks

MARINADE

1/2 cup fresh orange juice

2 TBSP sweet rice vinegar

2 TBSP fresh ginger juice

1/4 tsp soy sauce

1 tsp dark sesame oil

dash of umeboshi or red wine vinegar

1 (8 oz) package thin lo mein noodles or somen, cooked just tender.

1/2 cup roasted peanuts

Orange zest strips

2 TBSP minced fresh cilantro or mint

Bring a pot of water to a boil. Cook the carrot, snow peas and daikon separately in that order in boiling water until crisp, 1-3 minutes each. Drain well and transfer to a bowl. Add the green onions and ginger and set aside.

Prepare the Marinade Mix all ingredients together in a small bowl. Pour over the vegetable mixture. Allow to marinate 30 minutes. Toss the noodles with the marinated vegetables and marinade, peanuts, orange zest, and cilantro. Chill before serving.

Fettuccine Alfredo

This version is without the high fat and calorie contents so enjoy....

Serves 2-3

1 cup pine nuts

1 TBSP sweet white miso

2 cloves fresh garlic, minced

2 tsp fresh lemon juice

1 tsp brown rice syrup

1/4 cup extra virgin olive oil

Spring water

1 (8 oz) package fettuccine, cooked

2-3 sprigs basil, for garnish

Place the nuts, miso and garlic in a food processor. With motor running, slowly add all the liquid ingredients, except the water and process until blended. Add water in small amounts to adjust the consistency, keeping the sauce fairly thick. Transfer to a saucepan and cook, stirring, over low heat just enough to cook the miso and oil, but not enough to turn the lemon juice bitter, about 1 minute.

Cook fettuccine according to package direction just until tender to the bite. Drain fettuccine; without rinsing. Toss immediately with sauce and serve garnished with basil.

Angel Hair with Bell Pepper

4-6 servings

1 TBSP avocado oil

2-3 shallots, diced

Sea salt

Small piece of dried hot chile, diced

2 red bell peppers, roasted over a flame, peeled, seeded and cut into thin strips

1 green bell pepper, roasted over a flame, peeled, seeded and cut into thin strips

NOTE: Roast bell peppers or fresh chiles by placing over an open gas flame or under a broiler and charring outer skin. Transfer to a container and seal allow to steam several minutes. Then gently rub the skin away with your fingers, removing all the black pieces. Halve the bell peppers, remove the seeds and slice into strips or dice, according to recipe directions.

15-20 snow peas, trimmed

Spring water

16 oz angel hair pasta

10-12 leaves fresh basil

Red bell pepper rings or parsley sprigs for garnish

Heat oil in a skillet over medium heat. Add shallots and a pinch of salt and cook until shallot is translucent, about 5 minutes. Add chile, bell peppers, and pinch of salt and cook, stirring 2-3 minutes. Add snow peas and cook, stirring, until crisp tender, about 2 minutes and set aside.

Bring a large pot of water to a boil and cook pasta according to package directions until just tender. Drain the pasta without rinsing and reserving 1 cup of water. Add the cooked vegetables and basil and salt to taste. Toss well and transfer to a platter. Serve immediately garnished with red pepper rings.

Soba Noodles

Serves 2-3

Perfect lunch for a hot summer day.

Spring water

1 (8 oz) package soba noodles

DIPPING SAUCE

2 cups vegetable stock

1/2 tsp soy sauce

2 tsp brown rice syrup

2 TBSP fresh ginger juice

1 TBSP brown rice vinegar

Garnish with thinly sliced green onions, fresh wasabi, or thin strips or nori

Bring large pot of water to a boil and cook the noodles according to package directions. Bring water to a boil and add 1/2 cup of water, return to a boil and add the 1/2 cup of water again, return to a boil and add the last 1/2 cup of water and the noodle should be done. Drain and rinse well. Chill the cooked noodles completely before serving. If they stick together, run cold water over them and let drain just prior to serving.

Prepare dipping sauce

Season stock with soy sauce and simmer over low heat. Stir in the rice syrup and ginger juice and warm 3-4 minutes. Remove from heat and stir in vinegar. Pour dipping sauce into small individual bowls. Place the chilled noodles in individual bowls.

TO EAT: Transfer the noodles into the dipping sauce, add the garnish if you'd like and eat the noodles. It's one of my favorite dishes.

Vegetables and Noodles with Kuzu sauce

Serves 6

2 small leeks, thinly sliced

1 clove garlic, minced

1 TBSP sesame oil

1 medium carrot, cut into matchsticks

1 stalk celery, sliced thin

1/2 head cauliflower or broccoli florets

5 cups sprint water

1/4 cup tahini or almond butter

2 TBSP shoyu

2 TBSP Kuzu

1 tsp sweet white miso

4 cups udon noodles, cooked

Parsley, to garnish

In a skillet, saute leeks and garlic in oil until translucent. Add the carrot and celery and suate 5 minutes. Add the cauliflower or broccoli and 4 1/2 cups of water, bring to a boil then reduce heat to simmer until the vegetables are tender.

While the vegetables are cooking, combine tahini, shoyu, an kuzu with 1/2 cup of water. Add the mixture to simmering vegetables and cook 2 minutes, stirring until all is thick and smooth. Taste for seasoning and add sweet white miso if needed.

Place noodles in a casserole dish and cover with vegetable sauce.

Bake, covered, in 350 F oven for 30-40 minutes until browned and bubbling. Garnish with chopped parsley and serve.

Healthy Mac and Cheese

Serves 5

4 cups spring water

8 oz quinoa macaroni

Pinch of sea salt

1 cup fresh peas, blanced

1 batch butternut squash tahini sauce

"tahini sauce"

This sauce adds nutritious cheesy flavor to the pasta. Cook 1 peeled and chopped butternut squash in 2 cups of water for 20 minutes. Blend squash and cooking water with 1/4 cup tahini, 1/4 cup sweet white miso, 1 cup grated mochi, and 2 TBSP umeboshi vinegar. Slowly add more water if desired.

Bring 4 cups of spring water to a boil, add the macaroni and a pinch of sea salt. Cook until done, about 10 minutes.

Add the blanched peas, Mix Butternut Squash Tahini sauce with the macaroni and serve. It's the mommy approved for nutrition and kid approved for taste......

Salads

To me, salad is truly symbolic of freshness and lightness. Salads provide a way to live mindfully with nature and our environment. There is endless range of cooking techniques and ingredients to explore to create the perfect meal or a side to any meal.

Chopped Salad with Ginger-Miso Dressing

This is one of my favorite......it allows me to indulge in lots of fresh, seasonal vegetables smothered in the delectable miso dressing...yum...

Makes 5 Servings

1 cup cherry tomatoes, halved

1 cup diced cucumber (do not peel or seed)

3/4 cup shredded butternut squash or carrot

1 cup sliced snow peas

3-4 fresh green onions, thinly sliced on the diagonal

Ginger Miso Dressing

2 TBSP brown rice vinegar

2 TBSP sweet white miso

1 TBSP shelled hemp seeds or sesame seeds

1 TBSP Extra Virgin Olive Oil

1 tsp brown rice syrup

1 tsp Dijon mustard

Spring filtered water

Several leaves of butter lettuce or red lettuce

Combine tomatoes, cucumbers, squash, snow peas and green onions in a mixing bowl.

Make Dressing Whisk together all ingredients, slowly adding water to make a smooth dressing, but don't thin too much or it will not stick to the veggies. Toss salad and dressing together to coat well.

Arranges the lettuce leaves on a platter and mound salad on top and enjoy....

Escarole and Collard Green Salad with Pomegranate Vinaigrette

Serves 6

POMEGRANATE VINAIGRETTE

3/4 cup pomegranate juice

1 TBSP grated tangerine zest

2 TBSP brown rice syrup

3/4 cup extra virgin olive oil

2-3 TBSP balsamic vinegar

2/3 tsp sea salt

Generous pinch of ground cinnamon

1 Head escarole, rinsed very well, hand shredded

3-4 collard leaves, rinsed well, stems trimmed, blanched, and shredded

3-4 Belgian endive, halved lengthwise, sliced into thin slivers

Seeds from 2 pomegranates (if in season)

1/2 cup pecan pieces, pan toasted, coarsely chopped.

Make vinaigrette: Place pomegranate juice, tangerine zest and brown rice syrup in a small saucepan over medium heat. Cook until reduced to 1/4 cup, approximately 5 minutes. Transfer to a mixing bowl, whisk in the oil, vinegar, salt, and cinnamon and set aside.

Place greens in a mixing bowl, spoon the dressing over greens to toss to coat. Transfer salad to a platter and sprinkle with pomegranate seeds and pecans.

Roasted Zucchini Salad

This is perfect for end of the summer....

Serves 4-5

1/4 cup pine nuts, or walnuts

2-3 fresh zucchini, cut into 1/2 inch sticks

2-3 yellow summer squash, cut into 1/2 inch sticks

2 TBSP extra virgin olive oil

Sea salt

1 tsp dried basil

Juice squeezed out of 1 lemon

2-3 TBSP balsamic vinegar

1 bunch watercress or dandelion, rinsed and diced.

Toast pine nuts in a dry skillet over medium heat until lightly browned approximately 5 minutes.

Preheat oven to 375 F, lightly oil a baking sheet and set aside. In a medium bowl, toss the zucchini and summer squash with a small amount of oil and sprinkling of salt and basil. Spread evenly on prepared baking sheet and roast uncovered 15-20 minutes, until browned. Set aside to cool.

Whisk together the lemon juice and balsamic vinegar, pour over cooked squash and nuts and toss. Serve over watercress.

Healthy Greek Salad

Serves 3-4

DRESSING

1/3 cup extra virgin olive oil

1 TBSP fresh lemon juice

2 cloves fresh garlic, finely minced

Generous pinch of dry basil

2 TBSP white miso

1 TBSP red wine vinegar

1 tsp brown rice syrup

Sea salt

Cracked black pepper

1 large head romaine lettuce, butter lettuce, or even red lettuce works.

10-15 cherry tomatoes, halved

1 medium cucumber, cut into fine matchstick pieces

1 small red onion, cut into very thin half moon slices

1/2 pound cheddar cheese (preferably made from raw milk) or vegan cheese coarsely crumbled

10-12 oil cured black olives, pitted and halved

Prepare the dressing

Whisk together all ingredients, adding salt and pepper to taste. Chill completely to develop flavors. Hand shred or cut the lettuce into bite size pieces and combine with remaining ingredients. Just prior to serving, toss salad with dressing and serve immediately.

Beet and Avocado Salad

Serves 3-4

3-4 medium beets

2/3 cup extra virgin olive oil

Juice of 1 lemon

Sea salt

Cracked black pepper

1 firm, but ripe avocado, peeled, pitted, and cubed

1 small fennel bulb, thinly sliced

1/2 very thinly sliced red onion

1 cup baby arugula

Preheat oven to 400F, wet a sheet of parchment paper and wring out excess water. Lay a double thick sheet of foil on a work surface with parchment paper on top. Lay beets on paper and wrap foil and parchment tightly around beets. Bake 1-1 1/2 hours, until tender. Cool slightly before opening foil. When the beets have cooled enough to handle, peel and cut into 1 inch cubes.

Whisk oil, lemon juice, salt and pepper to taste in a bowl until combined. Transfer 2 TBSP of dressing to a small bowl and stir in the avocado. Toss the remaining ingredients, beets, fennel, onion, and arugula with the remaining dressing and arrange on a platter. Mound the avocado on top of the salad and serve.....

Red and Green Cabbage Salad

Makes 4-6 servings

Spring or filtered water

1/2 head green cabbage, finely shredded

1/4 head red cabbage, finely shredded

About 2 TBSP caraway seed

MARINADE

3 TBSP sesame oil

3 TBSP spring water

3 TBSP white miso

2 tsp brown rice vinegar

2 TBSP brown rice syrup

Bring a pot of water to a rolling boil. Add green cabbage and cook until just tender, approximately 3 minutes. Remove with a slotted spoon and place in a bowl. Add the red cabbage to boiling water and cook until just tender, about 3 minutes. Drain and add to the green cabbage and toss with the caraway seed.

Marinade: Whisk together all the ingredients until blended. Toss with warm cabbage and allow to marinate, tossing occasionally, about 15 minutes before serving.

Dark Green Salad

Paired with the sweet dressing, this salad is really satisfying.

Serves 4

LEMON DRESSING

1TBSP soy sauce

3-4 TBSP avocado oil

2 TBSP balsamic vinegar

Grated zest and juice of 1 lemon

1-2 TBSP brown rice syrup

Pinch sea salt

1 cup fresh thawed frozen raspberries

4 cups bitter greens (arugula, watercress, endive, and radicchio)

1/4 cup walnut pieces, lightly pan toasted.

Make Dressing:

Whisk together all ingredients, except the berries, and chill completely.

Rinse the greens very well and pat dry. Tear greens into bite size pieces. Arrange greens on a plate and stir dressing over the greens. Garnish with nuts and serve immediately.

Grilled Vidalia Onion Salad

I love onions, even raw, the Vidalia onions are so full of flavor......this dish will have you think twice about onions...yum..

Serves 4

2 TBSP extra virgin olive oil

Juice of 1 lemon

Pinch dried basil or several fresh basil leaves, minced

2 cloves fresh garlic, finely minced

2-3 TBSP balsamic vinegar

2 tsp umeboshi vinegar

2 Large Vidalia onions, cut into 1/8 inch thick slices

Green or red leaf lettuce

Preheat grill or broiler, mix together oil, lemon juice, basil, garlic and vinegars in a small bowl. Brush onion slices on both sides with oil mixture and grill until lightly browned on both sides and limp, 3-4 minutes per side. Arrange the lettuce leaves on a serving platter and top with the grilled onion rings. Serve immediately.

Quinoa and Roasted Veggie Salad

This is a meal in itself, you'll love it!

Makes 4-5 servings

1 cup quinoa, rinsed well and drained.

2 cups vegetable stock, or spring water

Pinch of sea salt

Sesame Oil

8 slices of ginger, cut into matchstick pieces

2-3 shallots minced

1 tsp each dried marjoram and thyme

1 carrot diced

2-3 celery stalks diced

Juice of 1 lemon

2-3 medium zucchini, cut into thin diagonal pieces

2-3 parsnips cut into diagonal

1 red onion, cut in half moon pieces

2 red bell peppers, cut into thin strips

Several cherry tomatoes, halved

Soy sauce

Combine the quinoa and stock in a saucepan and bring to a boil. Add salt, cover and cook over low heat until all the stock has been absorbed, about 25 minutes. Fluff with fork, transfer to a medium bowl and set aside.

Heat 1 tsp sesame oil in a skillet over medium heat, add ginger, shallots and herbs and cook, stirring, until shallots are translucent. Add carrot and celery and cook, stirring, until vegetables are just tender, 3-4 minutes. Remove from heat and stir in the lemon juice. Mix into the quinoa and set aside.

Preheat the oven to 400 F and lightly oil a baking pan or shallow casserole. Arrange the remaining vegetables in the pan and lightly drizzle with sesame oil and soy sauce. Toss to coat and roast uncovered until the vegetables are tender and lightly browned, 20-25 minutes.

To serve, arrange the layer of roasted vegetables on individual plates and top with a generous scoop of quinoa salad, serve warm.

Couscous Salad

This salad is a complete meal in itself....

Serves 5-6

6 cups spring water

Pinch sea salt

3 cups couscous

2-3 green onions, thinly sliced

2-3 red radishes, thinly sliced, slices cut in half

1/2 cup cooked chickpeas, drained

2 Celery stalks, thinly sliced

2 TBSP minced fresh flat leaf parsley

1 recipe Istanbul sauce

Bring water and salt to a boil in a large sauce pan over medium heat. Add couscous turn off heat and allow to stand, undisturbed for about 10 minutes. Fluff with a fork before proceeding with the recipe.

Toss all the ingredients together with the sauce and serve.

Pesto Noodle Salad

Serves 6

1 pound whole wheat noodles, penne or fettuccine

1/2 cup extra virgin olive oil

2 TBSP white miso

1/2 cup pine nuts or walnuts, lightly pan toasted plus extra to use for garnish

1 cup lightly packed fresh basil leaves

2 TBSP umeboshi vinegar

1 tsp brown rice syrup

1-2 cloves fresh garlic, minced

Spring water

2 stalks broccoli, cut into tiny flowerets and blanched until bright green

Cook noodles according to package directions. Drain and rinse well so that noodles do not stick together. Rinse until no warmth remains when you run your hands through the noodles. Set aside and prepare the pesto..

Place oil and miso in a small saucepan over low heat and warm through for a few minutes. Cool slightly before combining oil mixture, pine nuts, basil, vinegar, rice syrup and garlic in a food processor or blender and process until smooth. Gradually add a small bit of water to make a thick creamy sauce, if needed.

Toss the noodles and broccoli together and chill thoroughly. Separately chill the pesto and when ready to serve, toss together the noodles, broccoli, and pesto with some pine nuts for garnish, serve chilled, or warm.

Noodle Watercress Salad

Serves 2-3

This salad makes a perfect summer salad.

1 red pepper, roasted over an open flame, peeled, seeded and cut into strips

1 cucumber, halved lengthwise, then sliced crosswise.

1-2 celery stalks, cut into thin slices

Spring water

1 bunch of watercress

8 oz small shell pasta, cooked, rinsed and drained.

Red pepper rings for garnish

Dressing: Creamy Sesame Dressing

4 TBSP toasted sesame tahini

1/2 onion, finely minced

2 umeboshi plums, pitted

Dash of soy sauce

Juice of 1 lemon

2 tsp brown rice syrup

3/4 cup spring water

Combine all ingredients in a blender and puree until smooth, slowly adding water to achieve a creamy consistency.

Desserts

Let's discuss our sweet tooth. Yes, we all have one, for me when my hormones are raging once a month, a bit of sweet and sinful keeps me sane. So what's to refrain from? We can be mindful about our eating habits and enjoy the pleasures of food as well. So let's dig in and see what we can create.

Baking Caveats

It will make your kitchen efforts so much easier if you can assemble all the ingredients that you may need before you bake. Preheating the oven prior to you baking is also a good idea.

When mixing the baking ingredients, use a pastry utensils, not your hands. You'll be cooking with whole grains and they love moisture and the oil from your skin is no exception. Refrain from kneading dough unless the recipe requires it.

Flour

Whole wheat pastry flour is mainly used. White flour, is highly refined and nutritionally does not make sense so please refrain from using. You can however, mix the white and the whole wheat together with semolina flour if you are trying to achieve a lighter texture and lovely golden color.

Mix the dry and the wet ingredients separately and then fold them together until blended. This helps to avoid over mixing, which results in tough dough.

Fats

To create some moisture in the pastries, fat is an essential part of baking. Conventional baked goods use milk, cream, eggs, butter, margarine, or fat additives, however, for our alkaline program, we advise either the extra virgin olive oil, avocado, or the grapeseed oil.

If you are seeking to avoid the fat all together, you can try using the applesauce or pureed, poached pears which will make moist sweet cakes.

Citrus zests to any recipe is a secret to add flavor to desserts that lack the fat content.

Nuts

Nuts can really play up any dessert by adding texture, fiber, and protein. I recommend pan roasting the nuts prior to use to bring out the flavors. Roast nuts on medium heat for about 15 minutes.

Sweeteners

Brown rice syrup is by far the best sweetener. This grain based sweetener is made from complex sugars, not simple sugars so don't affect your blood sugar levels as much as the simple ones. They are simply whole grains inoculated with fermenting agent and then cooked until reduced to a syrup.

Stevia is another new player in the arena of sugars, they have intense sweet taste, I recommend that you experiment with it to make sure the amount is right when you cook. Stevia is a naturally sweet plant, and the leaves are broken down into powers that are then used. Try to look for unbleached, which should have its natural color green, not white.

Agave syrup is made from the cactus plant and can be a great sweetener as well. If you decide to go with this one, make sure that you use the least refined, which tend to have a darker hue.

Finally, there is xylitol, which is a granulated sweetener most commonly made from birch bark. Keep in mind that this is intensely sweet so should be used in moderation. The only down side is the price as it is   quite expensive.

Fruit-Custard Tart

Serves 6-8

Oat and nut crust

1 cup rolled oat

1/2 cup whole almonds

1/4 cup avocado oil

1/4 cup brown rice syrup

FILLING

1 cup amasake

2 tsp arrowroot dissolved in 1/4 cup cold water

3-4 cups fresh fruit; sliced strawberries, halved grapes, sliced peaches, pears or apples (tossed with 1 tsp lemon juice to prevent discoloring), blueberries or raspberries

GLAZE

1/4 cup unsweetened or fruit sweetened apricot preserves

1/2 cup brown rice syrup

1/4 cup spring or filtered water

1 tsp agar-agar flakes

Preheat oven to 350F

CRUST: Process the oats and almonds in a food processor into a fine meal. Add the oil and rice syrup and process to a dough. With wet hands, press the oat mixture into a pie pan firmly. Bake 15 minutes and set aside.

FILLING: Heat the amasake over medium heat and stir in dissolved kuzu and cook, stirring, until the mixture thickens approximately 3 minutes. Remove from the heat and stir in vanilla. Spoon the mixture into the pie shell, arrange the fruit in a eye pleasing pattern.

GLAZE: Heat preserves, rice syrup, water and agar-agar over low heat, stirring constantly until the agar-agar dissolves, approximately 10 minutes. The mixture will thicken slightly, brush or spoon the mixture over fruit while hot. Allow approximately 1 hour for the tart to set up.

Chocolate Cookies

Makes approximately 24 cookies

1 1/2 cup rolled oats

1 3/4 cups whole wheat pastry flour

1/8 tsp sea salt

1 1/2 tsp baking powder

1 cup unsweetened shredded coconut

1/2 cup minced pecans

2/3 cup to 1 cup soy milk

1 tsp vanilla extract

1 cup brown rice syrup

1/2 cup avocado or olive oil

1 cup grain-sweetened chocolate chips (typically available at natural foods stores)

Preheat oven to 350F. Line a baking sheet with parchment paper and set aside. Combine all ingredients, except chocolate chips, in a large bowl until blended. Use enough soy milk to create soft cookie dough consistency. Fold in the chocolate chips and arrange in the baking pain. Bake 18-20 minutes, cookies should be moist and chewy and cool on the wire racks and enjoy.

Oatmeal Cookies

You will love these cookies!

Makes about 24 cookies

1 1/2 cups whole wheat pastry flour

1 1/2 cups rolled oats

1/8 tsp sea salt

1/2 cup raisins

1/2 cup coarsely diced walnuts

1 cup amasake

3 TBSP avocado or olive oil

3/4 cup brown rice syrup

1 tsp vanilla extract

Combine the flour, oats and salt in a large bowl Mix in the raisins and walnuts, whisk together the amasake oil, rice syrup and vanilla. Fold the ingredients and allow to rest, covered with a cloth towel, in a warm place approximately 1 hour to allow the dough to ferment slightly so the cookies will rise.

Preheat the oven to 375 F, lightly oil a baking sheet and arrange the cookie dough leaving about 1 inch between the cookies. Bake 15-18 minutes until golden, do not over bake as it is better to remove from heat earlier than later.

Enjoy....

Glazed Apples

4 ripe apples

1 cup unsweetened apple juice

Pinch of sea salt

1 TBSP arrowroot, dissolved in 3 TBSP cold water

1/2 tsp fresh ginger juice

Slivered almonds, pan toasted

Preheat the oven to 350F, cut the apples in half and remove the cores carefully. Lay apple halves in a shallow baking dish, cut sides up and sprinkle with sea salt. Cover and bake for 15 minutes until tender.

IN the meantime, heat the apple juice over low heat until hot. Stir in the dissolved arrowroot and cook, stirring, until the mixture thickens and clears, approximate 3-4 minutes. Add ginger juice and pour over the cooked apples. Increase the oven heat to 400F, return the apples to the oven, uncovered for 15 minutes to set the glaze. Serve warm, sprinkled with almonds, absolutely delicious!

Pear Coffee Cake

Serves 6-8

1 TBSP avocado oil

3 TBSP maple syrup granules

3 firm but ripe bosc pears

1 TBSP fresh lemon juice

1 1/2 cups whole wheat pastry flour

Pinch of sea salt

1 tsp baking powder

2 tsp ground cinnamon

1/2 tsp nutmeg, ginger, and allspice each

1/2 cup brown rice syrup

1/4 cup barley malt

1/2 cup unsweetened applesauce

Place oven rack in the lowest position and preheat the oven to 375F. Oil and flour an 8 inch square baking dish.

Drizzle the oil over the bottom of the prepared baking dish and sprinkle with maple syrup granules. Peel, halve and core the pears and cut the pears into 1/8 inch thick slices, leaving the slices attached at the top half of the pears. Place the pears, cut side up in the maple syrup mixture, drizzle with lemon juice and bake uncovered 15 minutes.

Whisk together the flour, salt, baking powder and spices in a bowl. Whisk the wet ingredients, the rice syrup, barley malt and apple sauce. Stir the apple sauce mixture into the flour mixture until just blended. Spoon the batter carefully over the baked pears, covering them evenly.

Bake about 30-35 minutes until a wooden is inserted in the center of the cake comes out clean. With a sharp knife, loosen the edges of the cake from the pan. Place a serving platter over pan and invert the cake onto the platter. Remove any pear slices that adhere to the pan and place on top of the cake. Allow to cool about 10 minutes before slicing. This cake is great when served warm.

Decadent Brownies

Makes 16 brownies

1 1/3 cups maple syrup granules

3/4 cup unsweetened applesauce

2 TBSP spring water

2 tsp vanilla extract

1 cup whole wheat pastry flour

1/3 cup semolina flour

3/4 cup unsweetened cocoa powder, organic

1/2 tsp baking powder

Pinch of sea salt

Vanilla organic soymilk or raw milk

1 cup grain sweetened chocolate chips

2/3 macadamia nuts, coarsely chopped

CHOCOLATE GLAZE

1/4 cup plain or vanilla soymilk

1 tsp brown rice syrup or honey

2/3 cup grain sweetened chocolate chips, plus 1/3 cup coarsely chopped for decoration

Preheat oven to 350F, lightly oil an 8 inch square baking pan and set aside

Mix together maple syrup granules, apple sauce and water in a medium bowl. Stir in vanilla, fold in flours, cocoa, baking powder and salt, mixing just to combine ingredients.

Stir the milk into the batter fold the chocolate chips and nuts until mixed well.

Bake for about 40 minutes for chewy brownies and 45-50 minutes for more cake-like consistency.

While the brownies are baking, make the glaze: Place the milk and rice syrup in a small saucepan and bring to a high boil. Pour over chocolate chips in a heatproof bowl and whisk to create a smooth, shiny glaze.

When the brownies are cooled, cut into squares and spoon glaze over each brownie, you can decorate with chopped chocolate chips for added chocolate....enjoy.

Watermelon Ice

Serves 4-5

24 oz seeded watermelon

1 TBSP lemon juice

1/2 cup brown rice syrup

Lemon slices for garnish

Place the watermelon in a blender and puree until smooth. Add lemon juice and rice syrup and blend to combine. Transfer mixture to a large freezer container and freeze. Using a fork, stir the mixture every 30 minutes until it is frozen, it takes about 1 1/2 hour to freeze. Once frozen, rake the water ice until it is loose and coarse. Keep frozen until ready to serve. When serving, garnish with lemon slices in individual bowls.

Candied Apples

Makes 6 apples

6 red delicious or granny smith apples, rinsed well

1 1/2 cup brown rice syrup

Coarsely chopped macadamia nuts or peanuts

6 flat wooden sticks

Place the apples on a tray, top sides down. Cook the brown rice syrup in a deep saucepan over medium low heat until it adheres to the surface of the spoon, about 15 minutes.

Push a wooden stick into each apple. Holding the apple by the stick, roll it around in the pan of rice syrup to coat the whole apple. Quickly dip in macadamia nuts and place on a sheet of waxed paper until it set.

Section 32:
Resources

Organic Meats:

www.greensburymarket.com

www.wildwoodfoods.com/Organic

www.organicprairie.com

www.localharvest.org

Kitchen Knife: ergochef.com

Pressure Cookers/Various Cookers: kuhnrikon.com

Nuts: Chestnutsonline.com

Nut Butters: http://www.futtersnutbutters.com

Natural Import Company: http://naturalimport.com

Organic Foods: http://www.rhapsodynaturalfoods.org

Weston A Price Foundation: westonaprice.org

Quality Supplements: https://wellness.mymetagenics.com

My website: alkalineprogram.com, bestlifeblueprint.com

Raw milk: Realmilk.com

Section 33:
About the Author:

Connie Jeon is trained in physical therapy, pilates, nutrition, psychology, yoga, women's health, functional medicine, macrobiotics, fitness, manual medicine, and electro-diagnostic medicine and much more. She's an advocate for health for her patients as well as for herself.

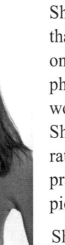 She believes that the health is our own responsibility and that no other person can better take care of one than oneself. She is passionate about the field of psychology, physical therapy, and nutrition as these three disciplines work collaboratively to make sense of the big picture. She believes that we are not parts that can be taken apart, rather that we are the sum of all our parts and refutes the practice of western medicine as failing to see the big picture.

She's looked to the eastern medical traditions as a guide to pull all the information she's gathered in her practice to integrate the best of the west with the east. She is a firm believer in the potential for human health, the premise for her work is that our bodies are already programmed for perfect health; it's our culture and behavior that is declining our health. She currently lives in Atlanta, Ga with her two boys and her loving husband. You can find her work on bestlifeblueprint.com

Printed in Great Britain
by Amazon.co.uk, Ltd.,
Marston Gate.